KEY CONCEPTS FOR THE STUDY
AND PRACTICE OF NURSING

KEY CONCEPTS FOR THE STUDY AND PRACTICE OF NURSING

MARJORIE L. BYRNE, B.S.N., M.S.

Curriculum consultant to schools of nursing,
Wakefield, Massachusetts;
formerly Assistant Professor,
University of California,
Los Angeles, California

LIDA F. THOMPSON, B.S.N., M.S.

Associate Professor, School of Nursing,
University of Northern Colorado,
Greeley, Colorado

SECOND EDITION

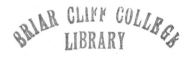
The C. V. Mosby Company

Saint Louis   1978

SECOND EDITION

Copyright © 1978 by The C. V. Mosby Company

All rights reserved. No part of this book may be reproduced in any manner without written permission of the publisher.

Previous edition copyrighted 1972

Printed in the United States of America

The C. V. Mosby Company
11830 Westline Industrial Drive, St. Louis, Missouri 63141

Library of Congress Cataloging in Publication Data

Byrne, Marjorie L
   Key concepts for the study and practice of nursing.

   Includes bibliographies and index.
   1. Nursing—Philosophy. I. Thompson, Lida F.,
1923-   joint author. II. Title.
RT84.5.B97 1978   610.73'069   77-26957
ISBN 0-8016-0920-8

GW/M/M 9 8 7 6 5 4 3 2 1

FOREWORD

The future of nursing as a profession and its ultimate effectiveness as a social instrument are contingent upon the degree to which it is able to develop an organized body of knowledge capable of predicting with accuracy the effects of nursing practice. This theory development is dependent on nurses who are not only well grounded in the biopsychosocial sciences from which nursing derives its theoretical base but who are also able to synthesize this knowledge into a unique nursing science. The focus of nursing science must continue to be on a practice-oriented, theoretical base capable of assisting the nursing practitioner in developing prescriptive goals with patients.

This book has been conceptualized and developed during a crucial time in nursing's history. As professional nurses accept expanding responsibility in the health delivery system, it is imperative that they take stock of their special contributions and talents. Man as an integrated biopsychosocial being is subjected to many stresses because of the supersonic rate of social and technologic change. Nursing's special contribution to health care lies in its ability to help Man to cope with his environment by providing holistic, continuous, and integrated care. Through the key concepts of nursing, well developed by the authors of this book, nursing's primary unit of concern is identified and analyzed. The primary goal for nursing practice is, and must remain, that of helping the patient to make maximum use of his adaptive processes in order to actualize himself as effectively as possible.

The key concepts of nursing described in this book, as well as their interrelatedness, will help both the student of nursing and the nursing practitioner to focus on a particular frame of reference based on a systems approach designed to place the emphasis on the whole man responding as a unified system. Through an understanding of these key concepts the practitioner will have a framework for gathering significant data essential for clinical application in the practice of nursing.

Mrs. Byrne and Mrs. Thompson have provided the nursing profession with a long-awaited and vital working model for assessing patient needs and predicting the effects of nursing care. The success of their efforts must be measured by the readiness and willingness of the practitioner to transfer this theoretical framework to the predictive practice of nursing.

Rheba de Tornyay, R.N., Ed.D.

Dean, School of Nursing,
University of Washington, Seattle;
formerly Dean, School of Nursing, University of
California, Los Angeles

PREFACE

We reviewed the many comments submitted to the publisher after the first edition of *Key Concepts* was published and were pleased with the reception of the book by the nursing community. Both the comments submitted to the publisher and the input we received directly from many nursing colleagues and students have been utilized to strengthen this second edition.

The first major area of revision includes a clarification and an expansion of the idea of Man as a set of human needs (Chapter 1). Many people indicated that more detail was necessary in this area in order to more fully comprehend the concept of basic human needs. Additionally, the expansion should promote a better understanding of the relationship between the basic human needs and the behavioral patterning of Man as a unified whole (Chapter 2).

The second major area of revision is the placement of the chapter on structural variables before, rather than after, the discussion of the stress concept in Chapter 5. This change provides the reader with a framework for examining the many variables that can influence the stress state when a specific patient is being assessed by the nurse. More important, however, the concept of structural variables itself has been clarified in such a manner that it provides a more workable tool for the nurse in daily practice.

The third major change is the introduction of the concepts of position and role. These concepts are inherent in the assumptions and beliefs presented on p. xi and are vital concepts for the beginning nursing student. Consequently, a new chapter has been included that presents the concepts of position and role at a rudimentary level. It provides students with a means for the examination of behaviors that are appropriate to the position they will be assuming and some of the more common problematic areas that they will encounter. Furthermore, it provides a basis for a discussion of the terms nurse-patient and nurse-client.

The fourth change is the inclusion of a chapter that examines the nature of the relationship that exists between a nurse and a client. The concept of a relationship provides the student with a framework for examining the scope and limitations of the nurse-client relationship as well as the stages that should be incorporated into any relationship.

These four major changes provide a more complete presentation of the key concepts underlying the study and practice of nursing. We emphasize again that each chapter of this book builds upon the concepts developed in preceding chapters. If selected chapters are read out of sequence, some of the content may not be fully understood.

In the first edition acknowledgment was given to a great number of people, because many persons, institutions, and organizations contributed in some way to the development of this text. Much of the original subject matter was acquired and winnowed from ideas aired while we were working with stimulating faculties and students in several educational institutions. We were greatly indebted to Lulu W. Hassenplug, Dean Emeritus of Nursing at the University of California at Los Angeles, who appointed one of us (Mrs. Byrne) to a curriculum revision committee that wrestled with many of the major concepts discussed in this book. During the preparation of the original manuscript invaluable assistance was sought and received from: Cynthia Barnes Aiu, A.D. Program, University of Hawaii; Marilynn Becker, California State College, Los Angeles; Sue Brueckner, Stanford–Palo Alto Hospital; Donna Freshman, Idaho State University; Pat Hess, San Francisco State College; Colette Kerlin, University of Colorado; Paul J. McKee, M.D.; Sue Parsell, San Francisco State College; Mary Ann Preach, El Camino Junior College; and Martha Seigel, University of California at Los Angeles. We also expressed our gratitude for the editorial consultation provided by J. W. McKee, Ph.D., and the invaluable assistance provided by our typists, Kay Niefert and Pat Detwiler.

There are three nursing colleagues whose collaboration has been an essential factor in the preparation of this second edition: Colette Kerlin, Associate Professor, School of Nursing, University of Colorado, Denver; Mary Ann Preach, Professor, Department of Nursing, El Camino College, Torrance, California; Martha Siegel, Associate Professor, Department of Nursing, California State University, Long Beach. In addition, I have been fortunate to have had Dorothy Karpowich, R.N., Ph.D., University of Lowell, Massachusetts, and Eleanor Drummond, R.N., Ed.D., Boston University, Massachusetts, critique this material. Last, the editorial service of my father, Dr. J. W. McKee, has continued to be an invaluable asset. I am grateful for all the support that I received from my husband and nursing colleagues during the preparation of this second edition.

Marjorie L. Byrne

A perspective for study
of the health care recipient

A PREFATORY NOTE

The nurse must have an in-depth knowledge of Man in order to develop an understanding of a patient. The study of the natural and behavioral sciences, which is an integral part of nursing education, provides many valuable but isolated theories and concepts that are relevant to Man's functioning as a united whole. The purpose of this book is to provide a perspective and framework for the synthesis and extension of these ideas in order to develop a greater understanding of Man when he is faced with a threat of illness. Understanding of basic human needs and the ability to interpret these needs through observation of Man's behavior as a unified whole will provide a basis for future study of disease conditions and their treatment.

The nursing profession as a whole has not aligned itself solidly behind any one frame of reference for nursing practice. Therefore our rationale for the perspective presented in this book has been made as explicit as possible to enable the reader to compare and contrast our approach with others so that individuals can identify for themselves the general framework they choose to utilize as a basis for their own nursing practice.

It is first necessary to identify certain assumptions and beliefs that we will be using to delineate and synthesize the content essential for nursing practice. The following statements will be elaborated on and utilized throughout this text.

ASSUMPTIONS AND BELIEFS ABOUT MAN

1. Man is an integrated biopsychosocial being.
2. Man is an energy unit.
   a. The amount of adaptive energy available to the individual depends on genetic factors.
   b. Tension is essential for "life."
   c. Each individual attempts to achieve a balance between utilization and conser-

vation of his energy; at that point he is functioning effectively and efficiently and is able to actualize himself according to his nature.

3. Man as a species has basic human needs that are common to all.
   a. Need imbalance can be inferred only on the basis of presenting or observable behaviors.
   b. Man as a species develops patterned ways of meeting these needs in order to maintain an optimal tension level.
   c. Each individual develops his own unique patterned way of meeting his needs; these patterns may vary from the norms for the species.
   d. The following variables influence the individualized pattern development and maintenance of the patterned behaviors: age, education/occupation, sex, relationships (primary group), religion, health, and cultural/ethnic group.
   e. Norms of behavioral patterning for the species provide a framework for assessing an individual and his own unique behavioral norms.

4. Illness interferes with Man's accustomed methods of satisfying his needs.
   a. This disruption causes an increased expenditure or inappropriate allocation of energy as he attempts to satisfy his needs in new or different ways.
   b. At times assistance from health personnel is necessary for the individual to meet his needs.

5. Man responds as a unified whole to any threat or change.
   a. All behavior has meaning.
   b. Behavioral cues that may indicate an intensification of the stress state can be identified.

ASSUMPTIONS AND BELIEFS ABOUT HEALTH

1. Health is a dynamic and fluctuating state.
2. The optimal state of health is not known.
3. The individual responds as an integrated biopsychosocial being; therefore, health cannot be compartmentalized as mental health, physical health, or social health.
4. Each individual is born with a finite amount of adaptive energy, the magnitude of which is determined by genetic factors.
5. The level of wellness that a person can attain and maintain depends on both genetic and environmental factors.
6. Healing utilizes energy, so that during this process that individual has less energy available for his usual activities of daily living.
7. The individual who is at a lower level of wellness has less energy available for activities of daily living, yet he is frequently in a situation that demands more than the usual amount of energy for adaptation as his usual patterns of behavior are frequently disrupted.

8. The individual has the right to determine the level of wellness that he will attain or maintain as long as he is not a threat to other individuals.

ASSUMPTIONS AND BELIEFS ABOUT THE RECIPIENT OF HEALTH CARE

1. Within certain legal limitations the individual has the right to determine whether or not he will utilize health care services.
2. The individual occupies several positions/roles simultaneously. He may be father, son, breadwinner, husband, friend, and sick man all at the same time.
3. One of these positions/roles is more central and pervasive in his response to illness; which one will dominate varies with each individual and his given situation.
4. In his sick role, the individual has both rights and obligations.
5. The individual frequently needs assistance in understanding and accepting his rights and obligations in his sick role.

As indicated earlier, these assumptions and beliefs provide the basis for the perspective and frame of reference for nursing practice in this book as well as the rationale for selection of content for the study of nursing. The list is not exhaustive but does include those concepts believed essential to an understanding of the practice of nursing in all of its aspects. It is expected that the reader will have questions about many of the statements made thus far; they should be resolved by reading this book.

After the reader has assimilated the basic assumptions and beliefs used throughout this text, the next step is the identification and study of the key concepts that are implicit in the statement of these assumptions and beliefs. Therefore, this book is devoted to the study of those concepts that will provide the baseline and unifying threads for subsequent nursing courses and the practice of nursing.

A WORD OF CAUTION

This book has been designed so that each chapter builds upon the content presented in the preceding chapters. Therefore, if the chapters are read out of order, the reader may be confused or fail to understand the material presented.

CONTENTS

Chapter 1

A NURSING CONCEPTUALIZATION OF MAN AND HIS BEHAVIOR

The very essence of nursing care rests upon the nurse's ability to perceive and understand the behavioral cues that indicate the patient's state of comfort or his ability to deal with the problems brought about by threats to his health. Ability to attach meaning to the patient's behavior is vital to successful fulfillment of the nurse's function. The average person is usually oblivious to many of his own behaviors as well as those of others; consequently, he interacts with and reacts to people on an intuitive basis. In order to develop those skills essential to nursing practice, potential practitioners must become acutely and consciously aware of their own behavioral responses as well as those of the patient. Nurses must develop insight into the variety of meanings that can be attached to a particular behavior in given circumstances and be able to predict the kind of response that will be seen as a result of nurse-patient interaction or manipulation of the patient's social and physical environment.

The natural and behavioral science courses that provide the foundation for a nursing major fragments the study of Man and his environment. Cellular, organ, and organ-system behaviors are understood in their singular aspect, almost as if they operated in isolation from the rest of the individual. Behavioral responses of families, communities, and societies are similarly organized for purposes of study. This atomistic content presentation provides the student with a sound body of facts and concepts that now must be synthesized and these interrelationships applied to the study of nursing. (See Fig. 1.) The nursing curriculum builds upon and extends the content learned through this atomistic approach by utilizing a holistic approach as Man, the potential patient, is studied in greater depth.

SPECIFIC BEHAVIORAL FOCUS FOR EACH DISCIPLINE

The term *behavior* is used to mean *response to stimulus*. Behavior is the action or reaction exhibited as a particular unit—be it a cell, a man, or a business corporation—copes with stimuli originating from either an internal or external source.

In the scheme of life, cellular behavior is perhaps the least complex or variable.

1

Fig. 1. Applied science of nursing.

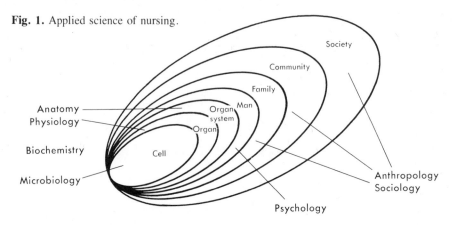

Organs are composed of groups of cells, organ systems of organs, man of organ systems, families of men, communities of families, and societies of communities. As progression is made through this list, behavior is more complex and variable. Therefore, it is proper and consistent to speak of levels of behavioral organization.

Behavior is a significant phenomenon for many disciplines in that their focus is on interaction between a structural unit of some kind and its particular environment. Each discipline designates its unit of major emphasis by identifying a specific unit and the level of behavioral organization that it has taken for its area of responsibility or primary concern.

Cellular behavior and the conditions under which specific kinds of behavior may be seen are well established by microbiologists. Organ and organ-system behavior is the focal point for the physiologist. Physicians often specialize in a particular organ or organ system; for example, there are cardiologists, urologists, dermatologists, obstetricians, and neurologists, to name but a few. Man's behavior as a unified whole is looked at more definitively by those interested in the relatively new field of physiologic psychology. Small group behavior, especially that of the family, is a unit of analysis when behavioral norms are being studied by sociologists.

Characteristic behavioral patterns of communities are identified by health educators in large metropolitan public health departments in order that community action necessary to deal with a current or potential health crisis may be made more effective. Some communities are characterized by lack of cohesiveness or organization and may be mobilized for concerted action only after a critical problem such as an epidemic has arisen. Others are well organized and respond conservatively, as evidenced by refusal to fluoridate city water supplies, prohibiting sex education in city schools, and the emphasis on private medical care rather than governmental intervention. Still other communities have responses varying from these two types. The latter type may be well organized but may have a characteristic liberal orientation toward health that includes a willingness to utilize all potential governmental assistance with community problems. Behavior at the societal level is discussed both by sociologists and anthropologists in terms of mores, value systems, and interactional patterns.

It should be clear that the definition of behavior is necessarily qualified by identification of the unit under study. The scope of each discipline's professional responsibility is delineated by this specified focus. The practitioner then develops an in-depth understanding of behavior at that designated level. He becomes expert in knowing the conditions under which he will see varying kinds of behavioral changes and in predicting behavioral responses; he knows what the norms for behavior are at the designated level and the action that will bring about desirable changes. It must be emphasized that the knowledge about behavior at other levels becomes a vitally important variable that the practitioner should use to help him to understand the "why" of what he observes at his chosen level of behavioral analysis. Usually, however, his knowledge of behavior at the other levels does not have the magnitude or depth of his knowledge at the level of his primary concern.

It may be well at this point for us to reinforce the purpose of the foregoing discussion and subsequent content of this book. When a student selects a career in nursing, he or she is selecting a specific behavioral level for focus and an area of primary concern for practice. Unfortunately, most nurses have been unable to define explicitly their central or unique professional responsibility and, moreover, the peripheral aspects of their role have historically been indistinct. New auxiliary roles have been developed to assist with nursing care, and there has resulted a movement for nurses to provide medically oriented rather than nursing oriented service to the patient. The dilemma with which the nursing profession is faced was very clearly presented by Brown[1] in 1948, by Bridgman[2] in 1952, Lysaught[3] in 1970, and again reinforced by Jelinek[4] in 1976. Brown strongly emphasized that: " . . . The nursing profession, collectively and individually, must take a positive position concerning itself and the significance of its functions."[1] The Jelinek report indicated that what was true in 1948 is still true today. Therefore, this text is designed to assist nurses in formulating their thoughts and thus to enable them to speak more clearly concerning the nature of the contribution made by the nurse practitioner in the delivery of health service in this country.

A FOCUS FOR NURSING

The nurse's primary unit of analysis is *Man as a unified whole.* * In understanding Man in this manner, the nurse must integrate facts and concepts from each of the

---

*While this book is focused on the individual as the nurse's unit of analysis, the student will learn to assess families and groups of patients as he progresses through the nursing curriculum. The principles remain the same. The basic concepts provided in this book will enable the student to move into more complex analyses involving several individuals.

Fig. 2. Levels of behavioral organization.

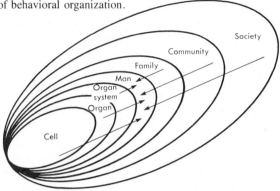

other levels of behavioral organization into a consideration of Man as a unified whole. Man cannot be understood out of context of the subordinate systems of which he is composed (cell, organ, and organ systems) or the superordinate systems in which he exists (the family, community, and society). (See Fig. 2.)

No one will deny that Man operates as a totality, yet, in practice, violation of this concept is often reflected in the attitude and orientation shown toward the patient and his care. According to Hall and Lindzey,[5] organismic theory evolved partly as a reaction against the prevalent custom of considering the mind and body as totally separate entities. It is more of a method of approach or frame of reference than it is a systematic behavior theory. It directs the investigator to take into account a web of variables and to consider the item of behavior that he is studying as a component of a system rather than as an isolated happening. They contend that an organismic theory is one that focuses upon the whole organism as a unified system, rather than upon separate parts, traits, or drives. Since the human being always functions as an organized whole, it is essential that the nurse adopt an organismic frame of reference.

ORGANISMIC BEHAVIOR

A definition of organismic behavior evolves from the following two beliefs about Man. The first belief is that *Man always responds as a unified whole,* not as a series of integrated parts. Man's mind and body are not separate entities. The mind does not consist of independent faculties nor does the body consist of independent organs and processes. Man as an organism is a single entity. What happens to a part affects the whole, and something affecting the whole affects the parts.

The second belief is that *Man as a whole is different from and more than the sum of his component parts.* The whole has a different configuration of behaviors than any of the parts. An analogy of water and its component parts may help to illustrate this point. Water is not the same as its parts. Its elements, hydrogen and oxygen, have different sets of characteristics and predictable responses. For example, each element alone will support combustion but combined as water they are commonly used to extinguish fire. Similarly, we see that Man, as a human organism composed of various systems, is something more than just the addition of his parts. He has a specific set of characteristics and many predictable responses to internal or external environmental stimuli. One cannot know, however, how a given individual will respond merely by knowing how his various organ systems respond.

The term *organismic behavior* can be defined as *those observable features and actions that reflect Man's functioning as a unified whole within the environment in which he exists.* Organismic behavior reflects the interrelated and interdependent changes that occur as a result of alterations in either his internal or his external environments.

Behavioral features refer to observable characteristics of the physical shell that houses Man. For example, one can observe skin coloration (bluish, ruddy, pale), skin texture (callus on hands), or perspiration (amount, odor, and location). Each individual has behavioral features unique to him. One individual will blush at the slightest discomfort in a situation, while another will only become "red in the face" when experiencing extremes in discomfort. Once the characteristic nature of the features has been identified for a given patient, the nurse has a series of readily assessable gauges for measuring his state of comfort. Some behavioral features are more specific to the malfunctioning of a given organ system rather than a unique individual characteristic. For example, cyanosis (blue coloration) of the nailbeds is generally recognized as a behavioral feature associated with malfunctioning of the cardiovascular system, and flushing is often indicative of an internal temperature imbalance.

Actions include any observable muscle movement as well as tone of voice, pace, and content verbalized by the individual. Observable muscle movements are exemplified by the individual who appears to skip lightly down the hall as contrasted with one who walks slowly with shoulders hunched, head forward. Similarly, one can contrast the content of the same verbal message received when the message is communicated by words spoken rapidly in a whispered voice and those spoken with moderate volume and carefully enunciated. All of these are actions giving us clues to the individual's response to changes in his internal or external environment.

Throughout this text, the term *behavior* will be used to refer to responses, incorporating both features and action, at the organismic level unless otherwise modified to indicate reference to response at a specific sublevel. We will be discussing behavior as a totality and will not attempt to subcategorize our observation as either behavioral features or behavioral actions. We have discussed them separately in the preceding paragraphs only to ensure that the reader would include both types of factors when assessing a patient's behavior.

Man as a system

Too often patients are viewed out of context of their home, family, and employment situations. They are diagnosed and treated with little consideration of influences from their accustomed environments. A person does not divest himself of all external influences just by walking through the doors of an institution, be it a school, an industrial plant, or a hospital. Yet nurses are often guilty of treating an individual as though he were a totally isolated, independent system, so it is necessary to explore the concept of a system in greater depth.

For purposes of this discussion we will utilize Buckley's definition of a system. "A whole which functions as a whole by virtue of the interdependence of its parts is called a system."[6] A unit qualifying as a system has a common or unifying purpose, boundaries, interrelated and interdependent parts. In anatomy and physiology the cardiovascular structure qualifies as a system for study, and the family is one system studied in sociology.

Analysis of any given system must include consideration of whether it is an open or closed system. A closed system is one that is self-contained, totally isolated, and therefore not affected by any changes outside its boundaries. Consideration of the heart and vascular system of the body in this category is obviously an inaccurate, although popular, concept. The accelerated heart rate resulting from a threat in the external environment is sufficient to demonstrate the error. A cell that exists in spore form that is not affected by temperature, moisture, or chemical changes in the environment might be considered a "closed" system. However, the notion of a closed system has little relevance in the study of Man.

An open system is one that is directly affected by happenings or changes in other systems. Man can be conceptualized as being constituted of a set of open systems who as a unified whole exists as an open system in his world. The interrelatedness and interdependency of two of Man's subsystems are easily demonstrated by the fact that an increase in circulating blood volume will result in an increased urinary output. Applying the same principle, a disagreement at the dinner table may well result in one member suffering indigestion as the family, the superordinate system in which he exists, exerts stressful stimuli on his digestive tract, which is one of his subsystems. Conversely, a father who has a headache may behave in such a way that the family interactions at the dinner table may be characterized by less free-flowing conversation and a lack of the usual good humor.

Although Man is continuously dealing with stimuli of both an internal and external nature, the changes will not necessarily be identifiable by the nurse when making a nursing assessment of a given patient. A change or response to stimuli in any one of the subsystems of which Man is composed can automatically bring about a corresponding change in the other subsystems and a potential for change that is observable. (See Fig. 3.)

There is only a *potential* for change in the configuration of the whole because Man's subsystems have automatic regulatory mechanisms that tend to maintain internal constancy; often, therefore, there is no observable behavioral change at the organismic level. The counteractivity that corrects the undesirable deviation often proceeds in an oscillating fashion. The restorative process consists of a series of pulls or pulls and pushes, like the swing of a pendulum that gradually approximates the center of gravity position. (See Fig. 4.) Occasionally there is an under- or over-

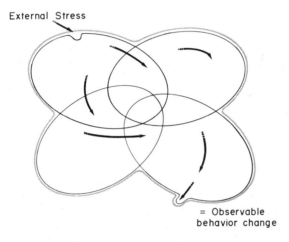

External Stress

= Observable
behavior change

Fig. 3. Observable behavioral change in response to a stressor. The gray outer line indicates behavior seen at organismic level reflecting a multitude of changes at the subsystem level when external stimuli are present.

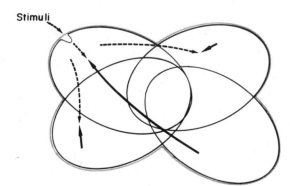

Stimuli

Fig. 4. No observable behavioral change in response to a stressor.

correction, and consequently some manifestations of the underlying activity can be observed by the nurse.

Man's subsystems, for example, maintain a fairly constant internal temperature while adjusting to a wide range in external environmental temperatures. There may or may not be evidence of this process or observable behavioral changes. In cases of exposure to colder weather, the body's heat production and preserving mechanisms are set in motion. The metabolic rate is increased, using more of the body's fuel and thereby generating heat. Shivering, a muscular activity with heat as a by-product, may be observed at the organismic level. If the increase in heat production continues indefinitely, the internal temperature would continue to rise above the safe upper limits and death could occur. The body's automatic regulatory mechanisms will effect a countering action, which will slow the metabolic rate at the point where internal production balances the loss to the colder external environment.

In conclusion, we see that Man as a human organism has a variety of automatic physiochemical regulatory mechanisms. These homeostatic mechanisms tend to maintain internal constancy by containing the changes occurring within specified limits.[7] Only if there is a malfunctioning of the homeostatic mechanisms or if they are overpowered by the number or intensity of the stimuli will changes be seen in the organismic behavior reflecting the underlying processes. Moreover, Man is influenced by his family, peer groups, and the community and society in which he exists. Therefore, a steady state exists when Man has an internal constancy and is in harmony with the world in which he exists.

Man as an energy unit

Man, as a unified holistic being, is in constant interaction with his universe and is composed of subsystems that are in a constant state of flux. As such, there is an ongoing energy exchange within Man as well as between Man and his environment. The goal of a healthy person is not simply to discharge or conserve energy but to attain an optimal balance between utilization and conservation of energy. Psychologists refer to Man's "psychic" energy. Dr. Hans Selye, a physiologist, has coined the term *adaptation* energy for that consumed during continued adaptive work to indicate that it is something different from the caloric energy we receive from food.[8] That Man is an energy unit is not debated, but rather the specific nature of the unit of energy remains to be defined.

The nurse is concerned with care and comfort of the patient and, consequently, must be concerned with the patient's adaptive energy. For our purposes we hypothesize that Man is an energy unit and that his energy is finite. In other words, each man has a given potential amount of adaptive energy; when this supply is exhausted, he will die. All life processes utilize energy. The amount of potential adaptive energy varies from individual to individual. Some of Man's energy is readily accessible and some of it is held in a reserve energy bank. Each man maintains a balance between the conservation and utilization of energy optimal for his functioning in life.

Continuing our hypothesis, there appears to be in each individual a built-in governor so that at a certain point any given part may either slow down its action or draw on the readily accessible energy from other parts in an attempt to run on the accessible rather than the reserve fund of energy. There is an attempt to equalize the energy expenditure for the overall system to maintain the energy utilization/conservation balance without drawing on the reserves. When the entire system's readily accessible energy has been used up, the reserve bank can be tapped. At this point, signs of exhaustion become manifest and the effectiveness and efficiency of the entire system decreases. This will be discussed in greater detail in Chapters 2 and 3.

The concept of energy utilization-conservation balance is an abstraction and as such cannot be pinpointed in concrete realities. However, it is present when a person is effectively and efficiently coping with his environment and actualizing himself according to his nature.

Energy redistribution, with its potential for imbalance, is an ongoing phenomenon in daily life. Energy imbalance for the healthy person usually results from external environmental changes, but for the ill person, it often results from both internal and external environmental interferences. The patient is a human organism having difficulty in his attempt to maintain stability with an ever changing internal and external environment. Only by achieving and maintaining stability or a steady state as a unified whole can Man cope with both the diseased part and the world in which he exists.

Goal of Man as a system

Now that the notion of Man as an energy unit has been introduced we are in a position to make a more comprehensive definition of the term *steady state,* which we identify as the common or unifying purpose of Man as a unit (p. 6). The *steady state* is that *state existing when energy is allocated in such a way that Man is freed to actualize himself according to his nature, maintained by effective and efficient activities of the regulatory processes at all behavioral levels.* In other words, the steady state exists when Man has an internal constancy and is in harmony with the environment in which he exists. Neither the automatic physiochemical behaviors nor the voluntary self-regulating behaviors alone will maintain the steady state. Only the total effect of their combined efforts results in maintenance of the all-encompassing steady state.

We believe that this definition of the steady state is unique to Man because the notion of self-actualization encompasses the belief that Man as a human being has a reason ''to be'' other than just existing. Animals exist; they have a code for survival, but it is doubtful that life or death matters to them. On the other hand, the humanness of Man is the fact that life does have meaning other than just existence.

Each person determines how he will best utilize his resources so that he has an inner peace; each person comes to terms with life by utilizing his potential as a biopsychosocial being so that he experiences the ''joy of life.'' For some this will take the form of a spiritual nature, for others communication through production of an artistic or literary work, and still others the sense of pride of workmanship, or any combination of these or other avenues. All of us seek to express our ''selves'' according to our natures in a way that gives us a sense of accomplishment and fulfillment. Self-actualization is viewed as the goal of Man as an integrated behavioral unit. Thus the notion of self-actualization is an integral part of the steady state definition for Man as a human being.

Man as a set of human needs

That there are certain needs common to all Men is a well-accepted idea. A review of the literature, however, reveals that there is no one taxonomy or classification of needs that has received total or even general acceptance. Murray[9] has probably developed the most exhaustive and detailed classification of needs, while Lewin[10] suggested that the word *needs* should be deleted from usage. Some authors talk about physiologic needs and others about psychologic needs. Still others will use a different label for the same need. Maslow[10] has probably moved the closest to implementation of the organismic viewpoint with his discussion of a need hierarchy.

Maslow considers Man's response to his needs as an integrated behavioral unit by examining the web of relationships between the various needs and the circumstances under which they would be aroused. He contends that, as a functioning whole, Man would give more credence to those needs most crucial to his immediate survival, postponing gratification of those considered to be less critical at that time. Maslow's need hierarchy from those most critical for survival to those less critical is as follows: (1) physiologic needs, (2) safety needs, (3) belonging and love needs, (4) need for social esteem, and (5) need for self-actualization.[11] According to Maslow's generalizations for Man as a species, if a person is extremely thirsty and dehydrated, he may be willing to put himself, as a whole, in jeopardy in order to obtain the necessary water. A teenager may join a gang to satisfy his need for belonging but risk rejection by the group if he thinks that he may get into a street fight and be injured (safety need). An artist who gives up his painting, which is meeting his self-actualization need, to take a conventional blue-collar job in order to keep the love of the girl he desires is demonstrating subordination of the self-actualization need to the love and belonging need. Maslow indicates that needs arrange themselves in a hierarchic order; those more fundamental to Man's immediate survival must be satisfied before those higher on the ladder can be accommodated.

The foregoing has been a general overview of the many ways of viewing needs. We have purposefully pointed out the wide divergence in the use of the term *needs* and have included Maslow's ideas in some detail because his work has been widely utilized by nursing programs. However, all the ideas presented have limitations in their application to nursing. None provides a means for integrating the knowledge of the body's automatic regulatory processes with the knowledge of patterns of behavior used by Man as a whole; none provides for the linkage between organismic behaviors used consistently to supplement and complement the subsystem's physical-chemical behaviors as Man carries out his activities of daily living.

A more comprehensive approach to the concept of needs is essential for the study of Man's behavior by nursing students. To provide this comprehensiveness, Man as a system can be conceptualized as being constituted of a set of subsystems identified as basic human needs. The term *needs,* modified by the words *basic human,* has a very special connotation that makes the concept more useful for the study of behavior of Man who is a potential patient. However, this concept of basic human needs cannot be condensed into a single sentence definition; it must be viewed as a multidimensional or multifaceted concept. (This does not negate the fact that a set of basic human needs will be identified or labeled for study using only one facet of the multidimensional concept.)

The basic human need concept suggested by the authors encompasses the following components, which are illustrated in Fig. 5.

Fig. 5. A basic human need concept.

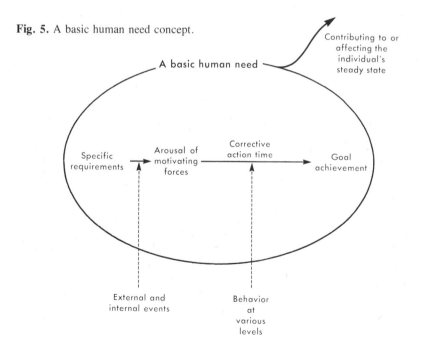

1. Inherent in the delineation of each basic human need is the fact that there are specific requirements of some sort necessary for survival.
2. These requirements become motivating forces when internal or external events cause a variation in either the quality or quantity of the requirements.
3. Arousal of these motivating forces impels behavior at various levels to correct the deviation when the deviation exceeds certain limits.
4. The specific nature and direction of the corrective behaviors is determined by the contribution that each need makes to Man as a whole.
5. This contribution can be defined as the goal that is achieved when the specific requirements are sustained within certain parameters.
6. A need imbalance occurs when there is a lag time between the arousal of the motivating forces and achievement of the need's goals.
7. Each need contributes in part to Man's stability as a unified whole and cannot be considered a separate autonomous unit.

This concept of basic human needs provides the basis for a logical and sequential study of the voluntary and deliberative behaviors used by Man as he goes about his activities of daily living in context with information about his automatic regulatory processes activated simultaneously. Furthermore, this need concept avoids the dichotomy between physiologic and psychologic needs, since each basic human need has a physiologic, psychologic, and social aspect to it. (You will note that this is a departure from Maslow's needs model.)

Since there is no one classification of needs that has received widespread acceptance, even within nursing educational programs, the authors have arbitrarily selected and defined the following set of basic human needs: (1) physical integrity, (2) affiliative, (3) activity-rest, (4) ingestive, (5) eliminative, (6) respiratory, and (7) sexual. This set of basic human needs represents a classification of motivating forces in their least complex and most rudimentary form. These seven basic needs are all viewed on an equal par because each plays, in some way, an indispensable part in maintaining the steady state. (This is also a departure from Maslow's model.)

Fig. 6 illustrates the notion that Man as a whole is constituted of a set of basic human needs. Man's steady state is dependent upon the balance that is achieved both within and among each of the basic human needs. Each need is an integral part of the whole; and when they are in balance, energy can be allocated in such a way that Man is freed to maximize his capacities according to his nature. Thus the *potential* for self-actualization is present when the steady state exists. (Chapters 2, 3, and 6 will consider maladaptive situations where the balance may not be beneficial for Man as an integrated behavioral unit.)

The box on p. 13 defines the basic human needs suggested for study. The need definitions presented include both specification of the motivating forces that impel

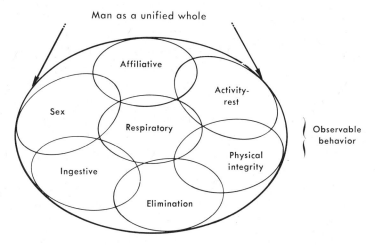

Fig. 6. Man conceptualized as a set of basic human needs.

DEFINITION OF A SET OF BASIC HUMAN NEEDS

physical integrity: those motivating forces initiated when there is damage or threat of injury to Man's anatomical structure itself. The goal is preservation of the physical apparatus of which Man is comprised.

affiliative: those motivating forces that impel Man to maintain satisfactory relationships with others. The goal of this need is to construct and maintain a position in social space.

activity-rest: those motivating forces initiated when there is inappropriate utilization of energy. The goal is coordination of behaviors that both utilize and conserve energy so that one can maximize resources without overtaxing them.

ingestive: those motivating forces that impel Man to replenish nutrients necessary for life. The goal of this need is to maintain adequate cellular nutrition.

eliminative: those motivating forces that initiate behaviors to rid the body of waste products of metabolism and substances that cannot be utilized by the body. The goal of this need is to protect the fluid and electrolyte balance essential for life.

respiratory: those motivating forces initiated when there is inadequate cellular oxygenation. The goal of this need is to maintain optimal gaseous exchange within Man and between Man and his external environment.

sexual: those motivating forces that impel Man to express himself as a sexual being. The goal of this need is preservation of sexual identity and continuance of the species.

behaviors and the goal of each need that contributes in part to the individual's steady state. This list of needs can be expanded and the definitions modified, but none may be eliminated without the probability of serious omission in the coverage of a basic need area. Now that a set of basic human needs has been labeled and defined, the concept of basic human needs presented on pp. 11-12 will be discussed more thoroughly. There are several major points that require elaboration.

The basic human needs defined for study are considered to be biologically determined and culturally modified. Each need has physiochemical requirements of some sort and each has a biologic goal that contributes in part to the overall stability of Man. Maintaining each need's physiochemical requirements within prescribed limits makes a specific contribution to Man as a unified whole and can be considered the goal of the need. Either internal or external events may change the quality or quantity of the required ''substances.'' These deviations become motivating forces or stimuli that initiate behavioral responses intended to resolve the deficit or overload so that the goal of the need can be achieved and the steady state maintained.

There are regulatory processes at the cellular, organ, and organ system levels that are attempting to keep the requirements within essential parameters and the needs in balance with one another. However, these physiochemical regulatory processes are dependent upon the give-and-take with the external environment as certain substances must be obtained and other substances eliminated. Imbalances in various parts of the body occur naturally and inevitably as various functions operate using energy, nutrients, water, or whatever is involved. The regulatory processes at the various behavioral levels are constantly operating to correct these imbalances. For instance, if the cells need more fluid, there comes a point when neither the body nor the cells themselves can provide the necessary moisture. Man must walk to the coffee machine or water fountain and obtain the liquid necessary to correct the deficiency. In other words, the body cannot satisfy all its needs internally; it must make use of external behaviors to secure whatever it is that the body requires. When the imbalance is corrected, the motivating forces subside and remain dormant until another deviation occurs. If the regulatory behaviors are effective and efficient, the steady state can be maintained even though there may be a temporary imbalance in parts of the system. (Chapter 6 will examine what is occurring when the activity exceeds the limits of the steady state.)

Man as a unified whole must interact with the world in which he exists in order to provide for the various need requirements. It must be pointed out that all the specific requirements and their parameters for each need are not known. For example, although the natural scientists are making great strides, the exact requirements of various vitamins (ingestive need) remain unidentified, and the specific requirements of the sexual need have yet to be determined. When the specific requirements are not yet known, we must depend upon the knowledge of the normal range of behaviors, at the various levels occurring under ordinary circumstances, to indicate the status of the motivating forces. This is one important reason for the emphasis on behavioral patterning, to be presented in Chapter 2.

Although some might question whether or not the affiliative need actually has a biologic basis, there is evidence in the literature to support the contention that it does.[12] Bowlby,[13] for one, suggests that there are neurophysiologic processes, through hormones and control of the nervous system excitation, that form the biologic basis for "attachment" behaviors of the species. These attachment behaviors as discussed by Ainsworth and Bell,[14] Cohen,[15] and Eibl-Eibesfeldt[16] fall within the realm of the affiliative need. The label affiliative need is used to cover a multitude of subdivisions often made and also to avoid the possible physiologic/social need dichotomy that is inherent when the term *social need* is used.

All needs are culturally modified in two ways. First, as a person interacts with his environment, *arousal of motivating forces becomes modified by his life experiences.* Motivating forces may be aroused by internal changes of some sort without change in the external environment or may be aroused as a result of external events. Thoughts of food (internal event) can initiate contractions of the stomach, causing a person to seek food or a means of satisfying that need. If an individual should smell freshly baked bread (external event) the motivating forces of the ingestive need may be aroused and behaviors initiated to satisfy the perceived requirements. Both internal and external factors that can cause arousal of the motivating forces will be altered or conditioned by personal experiences of people and by their expectations and standards of what is desirable or undesirable, good or bad, important or unimportant in various families, communities, and societies. For instance, initially only internal changes arouse the motivating forces that cause the newborn to indicate that he is hungry; however, in our culture, rarely does the adult wait until the internal status is such that his body requires food before he eats. Many people become "hungry by the clock." This may occur two, three, or four times a day. Exposure to desirable foods will often arouse the motivating forces of the ingestive need when the body itself does not require nutrients. Conversely, exposure to foods considered undesirable by a person may cause suppression of the motivating forces, a loss of appetite even though the body requires nutrients.

Second, it logically follows that *the behaviors used for goal achievement will be modified by life experiences.* One person will eat meat, potatoes, and drink coffee, while another will select fish, rice, and tea when he feels hunger. This point will be elaborated upon in Chapter 2. Thus what causes arousal of the motivating forces and the means used to achieve its goals are culturally modified.

It should be noted that all needs are not culturally modified to the same extent. The respiratory need, for example, is probably the least affected by Man's interaction with the world in which he exists. It remains the closest to its purely physiologic form of any of the needs since it is kept in balance primarily by the automatic regulatory mechanisms at the subsystem level; there are few voluntary or deliberative behaviors used by Man as a unified whole to keep the respiratory need in balance.

Each person establishes the priority that he usually gives to resolution of his need imbalances. The seven basic human needs are considered of equal importance because each plays, in some way, an indispensable part in maintenance of the steady state. A need imbalance was defined on p. 12 as that situation existing when there is a lag time between arousal of the motivating forces and achievement of its goal. However, at various times and under differing circumstances, one need imbalance may be more critical to the steady state of Man than another. (See Fig. 7.)

When there is more than one imbalance occurring simultaneously, the person himself, either consciously or unconsciously, chooses which will take precedence for his actions. His behaviors will be based upon the need imbalance that he feels can be tolerated with the least disturbance of the steady state. Conversely, he usually will initiate action to deal with the need imbalance that is causing him the most discomfort. *But the imbalance that a person perceives as causing the most discom-*

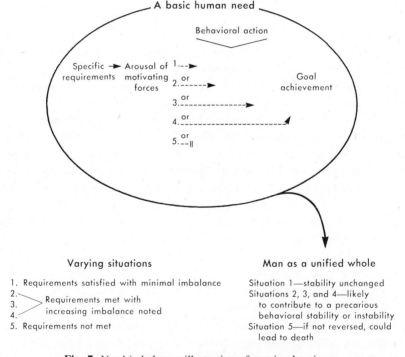

Fig. 7. Need imbalance: illustration of varying lag times.

fort in a specific situation may not be the imbalance that is most threatening to his behavioral stability. For example, if food is scarce, mothers have been known to starve to death because they gave all the available food to their children. In these cases the affiliative need took precedence over both the ingestive and the physical integrity needs. A person with diabetes may decide to skip breakfast fearing that he will be reprimanded for being late at the office if he takes time to eat. A diabetic crisis is, in actuality, more threatening to his behavioral stability than being reprimanded, yet he responds to the one *he* perceives as most threatening.

As a person grows and develops, a system of need priorities evolves that governs his daily activities. The need priority system is the usual way that a person ranks his needs under ordinary circumstances. Obviously one cannot sleep, eat, exercise, eliminate, socialize, and work all at the same time. For example, it is not uncommon because of work and social commitments (activity-rest and affiliative needs) for a person to go all day without eating or eliminating (ingestive and eliminative needs). The individual may sleep until the last moment and rush off to class or work after consuming only a quick cup of coffee. The hunger pangs and bladder spasms are ignored from early morning until evening in the rush of other daily activities. It must be emphasized that the latitude that a person has for determining his need priority system is influenced by the interrelationship of the following two factors.

One factor influencing the priority given to need imbalances is the *physiochemical requirements* of each need. Some need imbalances cause a person's behavioral stability to become precarious more quickly than others. For instance, the tolerable lag time between a perceived respiratory need imbalance and its correction is much shorter than that of the ingestive need; one can survive without food or fluids much longer than without oxygen. Gratification of the sexual need can be postponed much longer than that of the eliminative need without disrupting the steady state.

The ability to sustain the steady state in the face of a need imbalance is also dependent upon the *meaning that a person attaches to each of his needs.* Usually a person ranks the needs in terms of the importance that he attaches to them without conscious awareness. However, the priority system forms the basis for much of his decision making as he goes about his activities of daily living. Does he eat lunch or go to buy his wife a birthday present on his lunch hour? Does he go swimming even though he knows that he has an ear infection? Does he ignore the signals that indicate a need to defecate so that he can watch the end of a movie? A 20-year-old college student's affiliative need may take precedence over his activity-rest need, and he may become too involved socially to get the sleep he requires. Hunger may be tolerated in order to gain a slender figure if this makes the person feel more desirable (affiliative or sexual need). Thus the various decisions made throughout a day are a reflection of the degree of importance that a person gives to his various needs.

While the steady state exists, a person's need priority system may be very covert or difficult for the nurse to define. When behavioral stability becomes more precarious, the priorities often become more overt or discernible. One or two of the needs will be given more attention; they will become more dominant in the person's thoughts and actions than his other needs will. Observation of the choice and of the execution of behaviors enables the nurse to assess the priority that the patient gives to his needs.

The importance of priority of needs becomes apparent when one considers the illness dilemma. A patient's inability to adjust his priorities to the requirements of the illness situation can become a stressor for him. For example, an individual may give the ingestive need low priority in his daily life; the timing or type of foods and fluids consumed may hold little interest for him. However, serious pathologic consequences could occur if he develops a diabetic condition and refuses to take more interest in when and what he eats. Moreover, since the nurse and a patient may view the existing problem from different perspectives, their actions may well be governed by differing sets of priorities. A nurse may be concerned that a patient with a serious cardiac condition remain on the prescribed bed rest, while that patient, who has always been very bowel conscious, is concerned because he has not been able to defecate his usual two times a day using the bedpan. In just such a situation a patient climbed over the side rails and was discovered defecating on the bathroom commode. The nurse has the activity-rest need as top priority while the patient has given the eliminative need highest priority. Nurses must recognize that unless priority differences are reconciled, patient behaviors and nursing intervention may be in conflict. The many daily recurring situations in which the interrelationship of need imbalances is a crucial factor for determination of nursing intervention will be discussed in subsequent chapters.

The last point to be made in this discussion of needs is that a *basic human need is an intangible unit; consequently need imbalances can be inferred only on the basis of behavioral observations.* Assessment of a need imbalance is based upon observations of organismic behaviors as well as inferences about the various physiochemical subsystem behaviors. The latter observations are made indirectly through the use of clinical tests such as urine and blood analyses or through the use of equipment such as thermometers, sphygmomanometers, or heart monitoring apparatus.

All behavior has meaning. By attaching the appropriate conclusions to the behavioral observations, the nurse usually is able to identify the area of need imbalance and determine whether to intervene and, if so, what intervention is necessary under the circumstances.

If the nurse observes a person using accessory neck muscles to breathe and notes bluish coloration of his nailbeds and lips, and also feels the skin cold and moist to touch, he or she will quickly infer a respiratory need imbalance. The nurse cannot see inadequate cellular nutrition but does know that inattentiveness, lethargy, or crankiness may be manifestations of low blood sugar levels. A person may be observed nibbling frequently on various food items, or he may actually state, "I am hungry." Thus the various behavioral cues of a need imbalance may be very subtle or may be very obvious.

Absence of expected behaviors also may be a significant behavioral cue to a need imbalance. For instance, if a person ignores his food when it is known that he has not eaten for many hours or if a person has not defecated for several days, these observations should direct the nurse to investigate further.

It is not always possible to correlate positively a given behavior with a specific need imbalance. It is doubtful that the intake of several martinis is the result of a cellular request; other needs would have to be taken into consideration. The nurse will note also that the same behavior also may be satisfying two needs simultaneously while causing an imbalance in another need area. Examples of these kinds of situations will evolve in the discussion of behavioral patterning in the next chapter.

This basic need concept makes it possible to study the requirements of each need defined for study and to correlate these requirements with behaviors that, occurring at the various levels, lead to goal achievement when an imbalance occurs. Furthermore, this concept directs one to consider the interrelationships between the needs by continually focusing attention on their combined effect on Man as a unified whole. By studying Man's organismic responses clustering about each of the basic human needs, you will have a framework and background for assessing systematically the individual's responses when he becomes ill. The next chapter will be devoted to an examination of the concept of behavioral patterning that is a reflection of these clustered behaviors.

SUMMARY

We have now established that organismic behavior, the observable features and actions of Man as a unified whole, is a legitimate focus or level of analysis for the nurse. We have conceptualized Man as an individual composed of a set of open systems who exists in his world as an open system. We have established Man as an energy unit faced with the problem of maintaining an energy utilization-conservation balance optimal for his functioning in life. Furthermore, the goal of Man as a holistic biopsychosocial being has been specified as the maintenance of a steady state that incorporates the concept of self-actualization. We have indicated that there is a set of needs common to all Men and have presented a basic human need concept that provides a framework for the study of the regulatory behaviors at all behavioral levels used to maintain or regain the steady state when a need imbalance occurs.

These propositions provide the reader with a frame of reference for moving forward to an examination of the voluntary behavioral responses that Man utilizes in his daily living activities and their correlation with the steady state when he is faced with an illness.

REFERENCES

 1. Brown, Esther L.: Nursing for the future, New York, 1948, Russell Sage Foundation.
 2. Bridgman, M.: Collegiate education for nursing, New York, 1953, Russell Sage Foundation.
 3. Lysaught, J. P., director: An abstract for action, New York, 1970, McGraw-Hill Book Co.
 4. Jelinek, Richard C. (principal investigator): A review and evaluation of nursing productivity, vol. 1, Washington, D.C., 1976, U.S. Department of Health, Education, and Welfare, Division of Nursing, pp. 53-62.
 5. Hall, Calvin, and Lindzey, Gardner: Theories of personality, New York, 1957, John Wiley & Sons, Inc., pp. 329-333.
 6. Buckley, Walter: Modern systems research for the behavioral scientist, Chicago, 1968, Aldine Publishing Co., p. xvii.
 7. Cannon, W. B.: Wisdom of the body, New York, 1932, W. W. Norton & Co.
 8. Selye, Hans: The stress of life, New York, 1956, McGraw-Hill Book Co.
 9. Murray, H. A., and others: Explorations in personality, New York, 1938, Oxford University Press, pp. 291-292.
10. Lewin, K.: Field theory in social science; selected theoretical papers (Cartwright, D., editor), New York, 1951, Harper & Row, Publishers.
11. Maslow, A. H.: Motivation and personality, New York, 1954, Harper & Row, Publishers.
12. Harlow, H. P.: Development of affection in primates. In Bliss, E. L., editor: Roots of behavior, New York, 1962, Hafner Publishing Co.
13. Bowlby, John: Attachment. Vol. 1, Attachment and loss, New York, 1969, Basic Books, Publishers, Inc., pp. 210-234.
14. Ainsworth, M., and Bell, S.: Attachment, exploration, and separation: illustrated by the behavior of one-year olds in a strange situation, Child Development **41:**49-67.
15. Cohen, L. J.: The operational definition of human attachment, Psychological Bulletin **81**(4):207, 1974.
16. Eibl-Eibesfeldt, Irenaus: Ethology, the biology of behavior, ed. 2, New York, 1975, Holt, Rinehart & Winston, Inc., p. 490.

ADDITIONAL READINGS

Goldstein, Kurt: Human nature, New York, 1963, Schocken Books.
Kaluger, G., and Unkovic, C. M.: Psychology and sociology, St. Louis, 1969, The C. V. Mosby Co., chap. 4.
Menninger, Karl: The vital balance, New York, 1963, The Viking Press, chap. 5.

Chapter 2

BEHAVIORAL PATTERNING
an adaptive process

Identifiable themes or patterns of behavior evolve as Man copes with changes in both his internal and his external environments. He has a tendency to repeat those behaviors that have been found to bring about satisfactory results for him on previous occasions. Therefore, behavioral patterning at the organismic level is an adaptive process employed by Man.

PURPOSE

The maintenance of established patterns of behavior, to the greatest degree possible, minimizes the amount of energy the individual must use as he copes with his changing internal or external situations. The multitude of decisions involved in the basic activities of daily living that a person must make during a 24-hour period would be overwhelming if he had to stop and think about each one every day. Repeated use of tested behaviors under the same general circumstance is an energy-conserving process that frees Man to utilize energy dealing with less commonly occurring events in life. Without the use of patterned behavior Man would be so engrossed in the minutiae of details that his life in general would have little organization. The very process of getting up in the morning and dressing would involve literally dozens of conscious decisions, leaving little time or energy for work, study, or even interpersonal relationships.

By means of patterning his behavioral responses, Man attempts to maintain a steady state in his relationship to the external world as well as to his internal environment. Man orients himself as a human being in his universe through his patterning of behavior. Fear, anxiety, and anger are all natural human feelings often occurring when our life situation is threatened by illness. The individual's predictable means of dealing with the world and his place in it suddenly become very important. No longer can he take for granted the ability to walk, work, play, eliminate, eat, or sleep. If the individual can carry on his activities of daily living with as little modification as possible, it helps him to keep the illness situation in reasonable perspective. Indirectly, it tells him that his entire world has not fallen apart, although a part of it has been altered.

DEFINITION

In this book the term *behavioral pattern* will be defined as *a cluster of behaviors that appear to have a common drive or goal.* The behaviors comprising the cluster are those repeatedly used by the given individual. One could use the example of the variety of behaviors that cluster around hygiene to illustrate a pattern of hygienic practices. Tub or shower? Daily or weekly? Morning or night? Soap or partial soap? Preference in water temperature? Teeth brushed after meals, once a day, or not at all? Shave only on work days or 7 days a week? This does not exhaust the questions that could be asked, but it is enough to demonstrate the point that each of us has developed some very definite behaviors in the area of hygienic practices.

The basic human needs defined on p. 13 provide a set of motivating forces or goals around which the voluntary and deliberative patterned behaviors used by Man as he goes about his activities of daily living can be organized for study. There are identifiable patterns of behavior that can be correlated with each of the needs. For example, selection of food and fluids, preparation, service, and ingestive techniques can be considered as four patterns of behavior all appearing to contribute to Man's ingestive need.

Identified patterns are applicable to any society, community, family group, or individual. The specific behaviors that comprise the patterns will vary depending upon age, sex, ethnic group, religion, education, occupation, primary relational group, and health status. These variables will be discussed in detail in Chapter 4. If nurses have a good understanding of the generalizations that are available when considering groups of people, they can more quickly and effectively evaluate the behavioral patterns utilized by a particular patient.

Formation of patterned behavior

The process of behavioral patterning begins at birth. Crying is one of the earliest behaviors. The newborn infant who feels discomfort cries and the mother responds by feeding him or changing his diapers. The infant soon learns that crying produces the feeding, which relieves the hunger feelings. As the success of this behavioral act is reinforced, he utilizes it with regularity and predictability.

As the infant grows, he adds more responses or behavioral acts to his repertoire of coping behaviors. For instance, he no longer relies on crying alone to get the food when he is hungry. He may crawl to his highchair and try to climb in when he wants to be fed, or he may bang on the highchair table top when he wants food. He learns to grab for what he wants and to push away what he does not want. Crying, attempting to open the refrigerator door, and grabbing for foods may well be the responses that a 20-month-old child will use consistently when he is hungry. Eventually, he accumulates a core of behavioral acts that he has found ensure him reward or assistance in meeting his various basic human needs.

Once through the teenage period, a person generally has formulated the cluster of behaviors in each pattern that he will be using to satisfy his human needs. The individual has experimented with various ways of dealing with his life experiences and found the most successful and comfortable modes of behavior for him. Hopefully, the reader has already been exposed to such references in his sociology or psychology courses as Erikson's *Childhood and Society*[1] or Havighurst's *Developmental Tasks*,[2] since these writings are devoted to the examination of patterned behaviors at different stages of life or when faced with specific developmental tasks.

Lest it appear from the discussion thus far in this chapter that specific behavioral responses can be directly linked with a specific need imbalance, the point must be explicitly made that a particular behavioral response is *not* necessarily specific to a given need. The infant soon learns that crying, as a coping behavior, will cause the mother not only to feed and change him but, additionally, it will cause her to pick him up and cuddle him. He thereby learns that if he is lonely, crying will help to satisfy his need for love and affection. The crying behavior then becomes a nonspecific indicator of a need imbalance. Exactly which need area is involved must be determined by the mother. Is his diaper wet? When was he last fed? When was he last picked up and held? If she picks him up and holds him and he goes to sleep, she may well assume that he was just lonely and wanted attention.

Just as the mother must attempt to determine what need is motivating the crying behavior, the nurse must keep in mind that although there may appear to be a direct relationship between a patient's need and a given behavior, this is more apparent than real. In reality, Man responds as a unified whole; therefore, the organismic behavior is keeping several needs in balance simultaneously or may be meeting one need while causing an imbalance in another need area. An example of the latter situation would be the adolescent who persists in eating foods while out with friends (ingestive or affiliative need) that he knows will result for him in an allergic skin reaction (threat to his physical integrity need).

Established behavioral patterns

We have indicated that a behavioral pattern consists of a cluster of behaviors used with regularity and predictability when the individual is faced with a similar stimulus or need imbalance. It is essential that the nurse consider the regularity of the patient's patterned behaviors to better understand how the hospital or home environment and disease process may be affecting the patient. The basis for predictability of behavioral responses becomes more apparent when the two dimensions of regularity are examined.

First, the uniformity or constancy of the response to a given stimulus must be considered. The nurse will observe for the degree of *repetition of a certain behavior or behaviors*. When thirsty, some people drink coffee but never water, milk, or soda pop. Others will drink only tea or soda pop and so on, with the various beverages and combinations of beverages. Each person usually has certain behaviors composing his food and fluid selection pattern. Sleep preparation activity is another pattern about which people tend to be quite ritualistic. There are specific things that each person does at bedtime, usually automatically without nightly deliberation. A few of these recurrent behaviors are showering, setting hair, brushing teeth, setting the clock, letting the dog out for 5 minutes, reading a chapter in a book. After getting into bed and dozing for a while, a person may remember omission of an activity usually performed and actually get out of bed to complete it, since he has discovered that he will have difficulty getting to sleep if he does not do so. As the reader works with behavior and behavioral patterns, he will come to realize that the responses elicited by a particular stimulus are usually limited in number and kind by each individual. This holds true because most individuals repeat those behaviors that, for them, bring about the desired outcomes.

The second dimension of the regularity factor to be considered is that of *timing or cycling of the behavioral responses*. One may see a given behavior recurring at fixed times, be it during an hour, a day, or a longer time period. There is usually a definite identifiable rhythm or cycling of behaviors. In addition to the analysis of degree of repetitiveness of the behavior, the nurse would be considering the timing or cycling of the behavior. The person who drinks coffee may desire coffee only at breakfast, or he may want coffee with every meal. Even this comment may be too general because there are those coffee drinkers who want their coffee served with the main course and there are those who will be disturbed if the coffee is served before the dessert. Timing of sleep behaviors is often of critical concern to the nurse because of the difficulties imposed by regimented hospital routines. One individual may tell the nurse that he regularly retires at 8:30 P.M. and arises at 7 A.M. every day of the week, while another individual may say that he usually gets to bed around midnight and is up by 7 A.M. every day except Sunday. A night shift worker may indicate an 8 A.M. to 1 P.M. sleep period with a nap from 9:30 P.M. to 10:30 P.M. as his pattern. Disruption in either the repetition of responses or the timing of the responses can be very disturbing to the ill person.

Most people tend to limit the variety of their responses to those they have learned to use successfully in a given situation. A little further on we will examine the circumstances and what occurs when individuals become involved with alteration of their usual responses. Before then, however, it is necessary to indicate that there are persons who do not fall within the norms of the majority of the people. These are the individuals who utilize a wide variety of behaviors to serve a common purpose or goal. Variation in behavior of this sort can also be considered regular. This situation may be overlooked by the novice since the use of an extremely wide variety of behaviors is not within the norms for the population as a whole.

The nurse must recognize that for these few patients, the behaviors comprising the cluster are continuously changing and that this changing behavioral usage itself is ''constant.'' Actually, if one could make a longitudinal time study on this type of person's activities, a repetitive theme and cycling of behaviors would become evident. Unfortunately, this opportunity is seldom afforded the nurse who ordinarily interacts with the patient for only a short time. A person with such a varying response pattern can be far more disturbed than the average patient when hospitalized or in a situation where he is expected to conform to a regimented and definite set of behavioral expectations. The person who eats only when he is hungry and then eats only whatever happens to appeal to him, such as pizza for breakfast, has great potential for becoming upset by the traditional hospital 7-12-5 meal schedule with its arbitrary food selection plan.

Obviously, behavioral patterns do not always reflect or involve a conscious thought process. Successful modes or patterns of behavior are relegated to the background of conscious thought. Not much thought is given to food selection patterns that one has developed until the customary foods are no longer available or until eating them brings about undesired effects. A tourist traveling abroad may be dismayed by the absence of familiar foods. The individual who is developing a stomach ulcer may suddenly realize that his usual food selection pattern includes primarily highly spiced foods that one of his subsystems can no longer tolerate. The pattern of behavior will come into the foreground of consciousness only when something interferes with its use or in the event that the behavior does not bring about the expected or desired satisfactions.

Internal versus external environmental demands

Whether a person's internal or external environment takes precedence or focus for his energies is ordinarily determined at un unconscious level under usual circumstances. Man as a unified whole is usually more concerned with reconciliation of the demands of his changing external environment and takes for granted the functioning of his internal environment. This is possible because the body usually maintains or regains internal constancy through the subsystem's automatic regulating mechanisms without conscious effort at the organismic level. Man's relationship to his external environment, on the other hand, is dependent upon the control he exerts either consciously or unconsciously.

Nurses often see a patient whose concern for the external pressures is detrimental to the healing process. The illness itself appears to be of only secondary concern to the businessman who is in a state of panic because of a business deal that is about to fail as a result of the interferences of his serious illness. Similarly, focusing on the external environmental demands is the mother who signs herself out of the hospital 3 days after a hysterectomy because she is worried about her children, or the boy with a broken leg who refuses to use a cane after removal of the cast because of the fear of what his friends may say. All three have placed priority on external concerns rather than those of their internal environment and all three may have impeded cure and prolonged the period of recuperation because of their actions.

The external environmental priority is usually adhered to unless the malfunctioning part causes gross interferences with the person's activities of daily living. The internal environment is usually given priority only at such time as the individual learns that he is unable to function at all unless he will modify his activities to meet its demands. A teenager with diabetes may be counseled repeatedly about the need to monitor his dietary practices if he wishes to avoid serious complications, but all too often he does not follow the prescribed diet until after he has experienced at least one diabetic crisis. Only at that point does he recognize and begin to accept the fact that he must modify his food patterns to meet the internal demands and that these must take precedence over the external demands, such as eating forbidden foods when he is out with a peer group.

Alteration of established patterns

Once behavioral patterns have been formulated they do not remain unchanged, but rather the nature of the stimuli necessary for the person to alter his set ways of responding becomes different. Initially, every stimuli is responded to and incorporated by the newborn infant. As a person grows and determines who he is and how he fits into his environment, he will determine the manner in which he responds to stimuli and will become more selective of the stimuli to which he will respond. The adult has had a volume of life experiences and usually has oriented himself in his world to his own satisfaction. The majority of decisions regarding his direction and place in life have been made and he disregards many stimuli, judging them to be irrelevant for him.

The decision to change one of the accustomed behaviors in a cluster of patterned behaviors will depend upon many factors. A mother may tell her teenage daughter that her hair style is not becoming to her and be ignored. However, if a peer makes the same comment, the girl may immediately try other hair styles. Ten friends and a woman's husband may tell her that her hair style is "old-fashioned," but if the woman feels comfortable and attractive enough, she will disregard all the comments. If one student tells a teacher that she is making too many homework assignments, there may be little chance of change. Yet, if all the students in the class or a respected faculty colleague makes the same comment, the teacher will probably seriously reconsider her homework requirements.

The nurse must recognize that once a pattern or mode of behavior has become established, the individual does not readily substitute new behaviors relative to a given stimulus unless he himself determines that it is advantageous and desirable for him. Each individual evaluates the stimuli and decides whether he will alter his usual behavior by consciously or unconsciously considering the following factors:

1. The source of the stimuli
2. The intensity or number of the stimuli
3. The specific behavior or pattern of behavior involved
4. The importance attached to the original behavior

The nurse will utilize these factors in efforts to understand the response of the patient to internal or external stimuli associated with the illness.

Regardless of whether the cluster of behaviors is altered by free or forced choice, a greater amount of energy is used during the adjustment period than if there had been no change. Additionally, in a forced change situation, the energy utilized to cope with the change is greater than when the individual initiates the change on his own volition. People vary in the ease with which they are able to change their established behavioral patterns. The degree of flexibility in pattern alteration is a distinctly individualized phenomenon. Some persons are not disturbed when one or two of the behaviors that comprise the cluster must be altered, as long as the majority is not changed and continues to bring about satisfactory results. Other individuals become very agitated when any one particular behavior must be altered. Deletion of foods high in sodium content from one individual's food selection pattern is tolerated without an increase in tension or energy expenditure, while another individual becomes very upset when confronted with the same disruption.

This theory begins to take on meaning when one considers our hypothesis of Man as an energy unit and the relationship of energy utilization-conservation balance to the disease process. If some part of Man's subsystem is malfunctioning, energy is diverted from other areas to that part in an attempt to maintain or regain balance in that subsystem. As soon as the local, readily accessible energy has been depleted more adaptive energy must be made available, either from less accessible local reserves or from reserves in other parts of the body. When reallocation or depletion of energy occurs, all other subsystems and Man as a whole must function on a reduced level of available energy. This functional limitation often leads to a secondary imbalance for Man at the organismic level.

It is always well to bear in mind when evaluating a patient that illness usually precipitates a secondary crisis in the individual's external environment. Money problems, disruptions of social relationships, and job responsibilities are but a few of the problems secondary to the illness. A student who develops a respiratory infection manifested by a fever, headache, and general malaise may persist in working on an assigned term paper, and the energy thus expended can impede or critically interfere with the healing process. On the other hand, if he does not complete the paper, which was assigned 6 weeks earlier, his standing in the course is in jeopardy. This clash often results in anxiety and frustration with an excessive expenditure of energy in nonproductive ways.

Thus, when correlating the concept of energy allocation and disease process, it is necessary that the nurse recognize the conflicting demands that must be reconciled by the patient. The patient needs to reallocate his overall energy expenditure so that more energy may be available for the cure of the involved part, while at the same time he is required to expend more energy adjusting to the external environmental changes caused by his illness.

Adaptation versus maladaptation

In the preceding paragraphs the terms *adapt* and *adaptation* have been used. Adaptation refers to the process or utilization of coping behaviors by an individual when faced with new, different, or threatening stimuli. The reader is reminded that behavioral adaptation occurs at each of the behavioral levels: cellular, organ, organ system, organismic, primary group, or community. (See Fig. 2, p. 4.) The nurse will use knowledge about adaptation at all of these various levels while assisting the patient to adapt when established behavioral patterns must be modified.

It is essential that a distinction be made between constructive and nonconstructive adaptation if there is to be preciseness in assessment of the patient. Some behaviors will be assessed as adaptive and others as maladaptive. *Adaptation* is herein defined as *the positive, constructive end results, for the person as an ongoing functioning unit, that occur when adjustments are made to either an internal or an external environmental change.* *Maladaptation* then refers to *the nonconstructive or destructive consequences for Man as an integrated behavioral unit.*

There are many situations in everyday life that could be used to illustrate adaptation versus maladaptation. A familiar situation is the student with limited financial means who, rather than spending precious study time working to increase his income, decides to cut his living expenses drastically instead. His inadequate, low-protein diet results in both decreased attention span and lower level of energy so that his studies suffer. His behavior is maladaptive since he fails to benefit by his increased study time. Another common situation where maladaptive behavior is exhibited all too often occurs when a person takes two aspirin tablets and ignores his toothache, rather than going to the dentist for care.

Some behaviors are adaptive for a period of time and then, if continued, become maladaptive. Crying when injured is adaptive since crying serves as a tension-reduction and attention-getting mechanism. If the individual continues to cry and complain as the situation rectifies itself, however, the behavior no longer serves a constructive purpose. In fact, it becomes maladaptive since instead of drawing people closer to him, this behavior drives people away and lessens the chance for the assistance he is seeking.

There are two rather natural tendencies that must be considered, since they will frequently complicate the patient's adjustment or inhibit his adaptation. It is natural for a person who is uncomfortable or worried to focus on the present without much thought of the effect his immediate actions may have on his future functioning. The "here-and-now" problems may seem so insurmountable that he is likely to give little thought to the future. The patient may literally exist from day to day, minute to minute, or injection to injection. For instance, the person who has had abdominal surgery may not follow the nurse's instructions for coughing and deep breathing exercises even though he has been informed that these activities will reduce the possibility of complications, such as pneumonia, developing. Often patients confined to their beds will not have any appetite and will refuse to eat at a time when their bodies need an increased protein intake to enhance the healing process. Other patients have been known to resist the urge to defecate and later become very constipated, with the accompanying abdominal distention and discomfort. These patients will admit that they did not want to use the "uncomfortable" bedpan, with only a thin veil of curtain around them that allowed the fecal odors to permeate the two-bed room. In each of these cases, the patient was more concerned with the present than he was with the future.

It is also natural for a person to focus on the "involved part" to the exclusion of those other parts that he considers to be functioning satisfactorily. The patient will frequently have difficulty evaluating his actions as a total functioning unit. A woman may refuse to sign a permit for a mastectomy (removal of a breast) because she views loss of that body part as so traumatic that she cannot consider the fact that the cancer could spread throughout her entire body. This woman finds it difficult to make a decision that is positive for herself as a whole because the consequences for the involved part are viewed so negatively.

There are other situations where the individual's behaviors may have positive consequences for the "part" and yet, for the person as a whole, be negative. The individual who has arthritis (inflammation of the joints) may have very painful and "swollen" joints. The inflammatory process can be aggravated by movement of the joint, and yet the muscles used to control joint movement must receive some stimulation if they are not to atrophy (waste away). The patient will likely tend to limit the involved joint motion in order to avoid pain. Therefore, it is possible that when the inflammation recedes a person may be left with a nonfunctioning joint. Such people are "crippled" not necessarily by the disease pathology itself but by their coping behaviors used to avoid discomfort. In their effort to avoid discomfort of the involved part, these people often reduce their overall activity. Muscles in other parts of the body are used less, resulting in a general loss of muscle tone, and the person becomes weak and easily fatigued and has difficulty carrying out his ordinary daily activities. This individual is focusing on the "immediate here-and-now" problems and is not evaluating himself as a total functioning unit.

The extreme is reached by those patients who tend to evaluate all their daily activities as if they consisted only of a ''part.'' One man literally saw himself as a ''bowel.'' He evaluated his food intake not in terms of the basic four food groups but rather on the effect that he thought the foods would have on his bowel and, consequently, he had a very unbalanced diet. He also limited the amount of exercise undertaken because he thought activity made his bowel ''overactive,'' and he developed the habit of shallow breathing because deep breaths ''caused abdominal pressures.'' He wouldn't sleep on his stomach because of the pressure on the intestinal tract and, of course, sex relations with his wife were abandoned. It should be obvious that the nurse must assess both the degree of emphasis the patient places on the ''here-and-now'' problems and on the ''involved part.'' These very natural tendencies can be maladaptive since they can impede restoration of the steady state.

When making an overall assessment of the patient's adaptation or maladaptation, the nurse must question in her mind:
1. How does the patient view his situation?
    a. What priority does the patient give to his human needs?
    b. Does he have only a here-and-now orientation?
    c. Is he seeing himself as a unified whole or only as his involved part?
2. What are the behaviors comprising the patient's usual patterns of daily living?
3. What are the disruptions in his usual behaviors resulting from the illness situation?
4. Within the limits of the medical regimen, which of the disruptions in his behavioral patterns are actually necessary?

The following situation demonstrates how a patient may utilize maladaptive behaviors in his attempt to adjust to a variety of enforced changes in his usual behavioral patterns. A man with a broken leg in traction was faced with a situation where the majority of usual daily living behaviors could no longer be carried out. He was accustomed to sleeping from 2 A.M. to 10 A.M., but in the hospital he was tucked into bed by 10 P.M. and was awakened by 5 A.M. He had to use a urinal in a horizontal position instead of standing at a commode in his private bathroom. He had a limited selection of foods and the time of meals was rigidly enforced. At home, he bathed in a tub at night twice a week; here, every morning the nurse or nurse's aide bathed him in bed. He was accustomed to little social interaction because his work was with objects on a production line and he lived alone. In this situation he had frequent staff company, but his few friends were only allowed to see him for a short time after lunch as they worked from 4 P.M. to midnight. He was accustomed to sleeping on his stomach and now he had to stay on his back or side.

This patient purposely moved down in bed so that the traction weights rested on the floor, refused to have a bath more than twice a week, frequently refused to eat what was on the food tray, argued with the nurses when they attempted to get him settled for sleep by 10 P.M., swore heartily at them when awakened by 5 A.M. to have his temperature taken, and other such behaviors. The overall consequence of this patient's behavior was maladaptive as he was both hindering the cure process and driving the staff away from him.

The staff will consider such a patient to be grouchy and uncooperative unless they recognize that his behavior may well be a reflection of the disruption of his usual modes of behavior. This situation can be anticipated and the nurse can frequently modify some of the hospital routines so that they are more compatible with the patient's usual patterns of behavior. The nurses can modify food selection, timing of baths, visiting hours, and hour of sleep without interfering with the prescribed treatments. When this man was allowed to order special foods, given a full bath only twice a week with good back care twice a day, and allowed to watch the late movie on television and sleep until 8 A.M., there was an abrupt change in his overall behavior. When the nurse attempted to minimize the total number of patterns disrupted, he was able to accept the fact that his position in bed and his elimination patterns necessarily had to be changed in order to carry out the medical regimen.

SUMMARY

It has been indicated that there are identifiable clusters of behaviors that appear to have a common drive or goal, since people tend to limit the kind and number of behaviors they will use when responding to a given stimulus or need imbalance. These regular and predictable patterns of behavior evolve as an individual experiments and determines the most satisfactory ways of dealing with his particular life experiences. These self-regulating behaviors are used either consciously or unconsciously and contribute to maintenance of the steady state.

The nurse assesses the patient's behavior in an attempt to determine the particular need imbalance, since she knows that, as an integrated behavioral unit, Man's behavior may be meeting several needs simultaneously or may be satisfying one while causing an imbalance in another. The nurse knows that if the individual's usual behaviors for coping with his activities of daily living cannot be continued or no longer have the potential for success, he has two alternatives: attempt to continue the old behaviors that will meet with failure or substitute new behaviors. Regardless of the alternative selected by the patient, more energy is utilized in the response than if the usual mode or pattern of behavior had not been altered or disrupted. Continuation of established behaviors that will meet with failure is obviously maladaptive. New behaviors used to adjust to changes in internal or external environments may be either adaptive or maladaptive.

Nurses must determine the effectiveness of the patient's coping behaviors as he carries out his activities of daily living in the illness situation. They are aware that the external environmental demands will ordinarily take precedence over the internal demands unless the malfunctioning part grossly interferes with the individual's usual activities. Evaluation of the consequences or potential consequences of these behaviors must take into consideration the individual as an ongoing total functioning unit. In this way, the adaptive behaviors can be reinforced by the nurse and maladaptive behaviors can be identified and appropriate nursing intervention initiated.

REFERENCES

1. Erikson, Erik H.: Childhood and society, New York, 1950, W. W. Norton & Co., Inc.
2. Havighurst, Robert: Developmental tasks and education, New York, 1952, Longmans, Green.

ADDITIONAL READINGS

Child, I. L., and Zigler, Edward: Socialization. In Lindzey, Gardner, and Aronson, Elliot, editors: Handbook of social psychology, ed. 2, vol. 3, Reading, Mass., 1968, Addison-Wesley Publishing Co., Inc., pp. 501-555.
Colter, Rule: Theories of human behavior based on studies of non-human primates. In Kiev, Ari: Social psychiatry, New York, 1969, Science House, Inc.
Cummings, E., and Henry, W. E.: Growing old, New York, 1961, Basic Books, Inc., Publishers.
Erikson, Erik H.: Identity and the life cycle, Psychological Issues 1(1):1-75, 1959.
Scott, John P.: Animal behavior, Chicago, 1958, University of Chicago Press.

Chapter 3

BEHAVIORAL STABILITY
a reflection of Man's energy allocation

A person's adaptation can be interfered with if his expectations for nursing care do not correlate with those of the nurse. Should their expectations actually be in conflict, the patient's stability may be affected. Therefore, we will digress slightly to examine the most frequent reason for this confusion before launching into the discussion of behavioral stability.

CARE AND COMFORT

Nursing literature contains many references to patient "care and comfort" as the nurse's goal. There is a vast difference, however, between the lay connotation of "care and comfort" and the professional usage of the terms. Much of the discrepancy in defining the role of the nurse stems from this fundamental difference in the interpretation of these words. It is not a matter of right and wrong but rather that the lay definition arises from a different perspective.

"Care and comfort" to the nonmedical person usually denotes activities leading to or allowing less energy expenditure by the ill person. Patients are often enjoined with such platitudes as "take it easy," "relax," "rest awhile," or "don't worry." Mothers frequently insist that their children remain in bed without any toys while recuperating from childhood diseases, such as measles and chicken pox. They are amazed to learn that frequently more energy is used "not playing" than if the child is allowed to play quietly on the floor with his trains or blocks. Relatives sometimes are annoyed with the nursing staff when they discover that a patient has assisted with his own bath or has gotten out of bed while the nurse changed the linens. These relatives may be disturbed because they view having things done for the patient as a fundamental service for which they are paying. Unfortunately, some nurses also view "care and comfort" in this manner and indiscriminately do things for their patients. There are still too many hospitals where nurses or their aides give every patient, regardless of his condition, a complete bed bath every day.

The continuation of "doing for" patients when it is no longer necessary can be very detrimental to their progress. A nurse who gives every patient confined to his bed a complete bed bath may be robbing some of these patients of much-needed activity essential to the improvement of their blood circulation and muscle tone. Moreover, doing everything for the patient may reinforce his feelings of helplessness or of being an invalid. Activities performed for the patient must be based on a reasoned expectation of positive consequences. Productive allocation of the patient's energies must provide the rationale rather than the fact that it is a "hospital routine" indiscriminately followed by all in every situation.

We contend that the professional interpretation of the terms *care* and *comfort* must be in harmony with and flow out of the goal of nursing; that within the limits of the illness situation, the individual will be functioning both as effectively and efficiently as possible and actualizing himself according to his nature. This means that the nurse must be concerned with the overall allocation or apportionment of a patient's energy and not just limit herself to carrying out energy-conservation measures on the patient's behalf. The full impact of this statement will become clearer in subsequent chapters.

A patient may be allocating his energy inappropriately in an attempt to adjust to his altered circumstances. A patient may overdo his walking because he thinks that if one lap around the halls is good for him, ten laps will be better. He may then return to his bed and move as little as possible for the remainder of the day. In this case, both the timing and the degree of activity over the 24-hour period should be discussed with the patient.

As a result of an assessment and within the limitation of the medical regimen, there are times when nurses must purposefully manipulate the situation in order to increase the energy expenditure by a patient. The individual who has had abdominal surgery may be content to move as little as possible and to get out of bed may seem like an impossibility to him. Nurses know that there are many complications at the organ system level, such as lung congestion, thrombophlebitis, or lack of bowel activity that often occur if the patient is allowed to remain motionless. They know that these potential complications far outweigh the factors of pain, fear, and fatigue at the organismic level in this situation. In most cases, the patient can be influenced to tolerate the peaking of energy expenditure in order to avoid a prolonged imbalance should complications occur.

There are instances when nurses must purposefully increase the patient's energy utilization in order to keep him from a life-or-death emergency. Some diabetic patients must monitor their food selection, preparation, and service patterns if they are to avoid a hypo- or hyperglycemic crisis. In such cases, the nurse must hold rigidly to the prescribed food regimen and see that the patient adheres to these restrictions, even though this may involve disruption of his usual behavioral patterns and, consequently, increase his energy utilization. However, by minimizing the number of his other behavioral patterns disrupted, the probability of his incorporation of the required changes into his food pattern will be maximized. Adjustment to the required changes is more likely to occur when other unnecessary changes are not simultaneously demanded. Hopefully, as the patient understands more about his diabetic condition and its relationship to his usual life style, he will be motivated to accept the necessary changes. At that point, he will be able to maintain his internal constancy and will be in harmony with his external world.

The nurse must equate the words "care and comfort" with constructive allocation of the patient's energies, since equating them with energy conservation alone can be very detrimental to the patient's welfare. Nurses must become aware that this is not a universally accepted notion, however, and must keep the patient, his involved family, and friends fully informed as to the "how and why" of the necessary regimen.

ASSESSMENT OF ENERGY ALLOCATION AND ADAPTATION

Nurses are confronted with the problem of determining the adaptive status of each patient as he adjusts to changes caused by illness or potential illness.* They must have a method for logically and comprehensively assessing whether the patient is allocating his energies appropriately for effective and efficient functioning within the limitations of his current situation. Although the energy utilization/conservation balance itself cannot be measured directly, the behavioral features and actions that reflect energy allocation can be monitored. Consequently, *examination of the orderliness, consistency, and coherency of a person's behaviors will give an indication of the manner in which that person is allocating his energies and how effectively he is coping with his life situation.* These nursing observations are put into perspective by utilizing the concept of a continuum of behavioral stability.

A behavioral continuum

Man's functioning as an integrated behavioral unit can be viewed on a continuum. On one end of the spectrum he is operating as a stable, integrated unit and on the other as an unstable, nonintegrated behavioral unit. At various times and under differing conditions the individual will move back and forth between two poles. As he moves from the point of stability to instability, he is a precariously functioning unit. Admittedly, the scale is unrefined, but its indices will enable the nurse to judge how the person, as a unified whole, is coping with stimuli of either an internal or external nature. The individual's specific behaviors in and of themselves are not to be judged as stable or unstable; rather, they provide the nurse with

---

*Exposure to typhoid fever would be an example of a potential illness situation. A mother being prohibited from preparing meals for her family pending outcome of tests or the termination of the incubation period would be an example of a change caused by a "potential illness."

information as to his position on the stability continuum and the status of his adaptation as a unified whole.

When the individual is operating on the stable end of the continuum, the nurse will observe behaviors that are consistent, coherent, and orderly. The person's behaviors will be both effective and efficient and he will be allocating his energies appropriately. On the opposite end, the nurse can identify behaviors that are inconsistent, incoherent, and without order. The behaviors are neither effective nor efficient for him as an integrated unit. An individual in a state of panic, hysteria, or unconsciousness could be considered on the instability end of the spectrum. In between is the area of precarious stability, which is manifested by behaviors that may be either efficient but not effective or effective but not efficient. The individual is utilizing an excessive amount of energy to complete a given action. There is an identifiable distortion in either consistency, coherency, or orderliness of *some* of his behaviors.

The concept of an organismic behavioral stability continuum is illustrated in Fig. 8 by a man standing on a seesaw with one foot on either side of the fulcrum

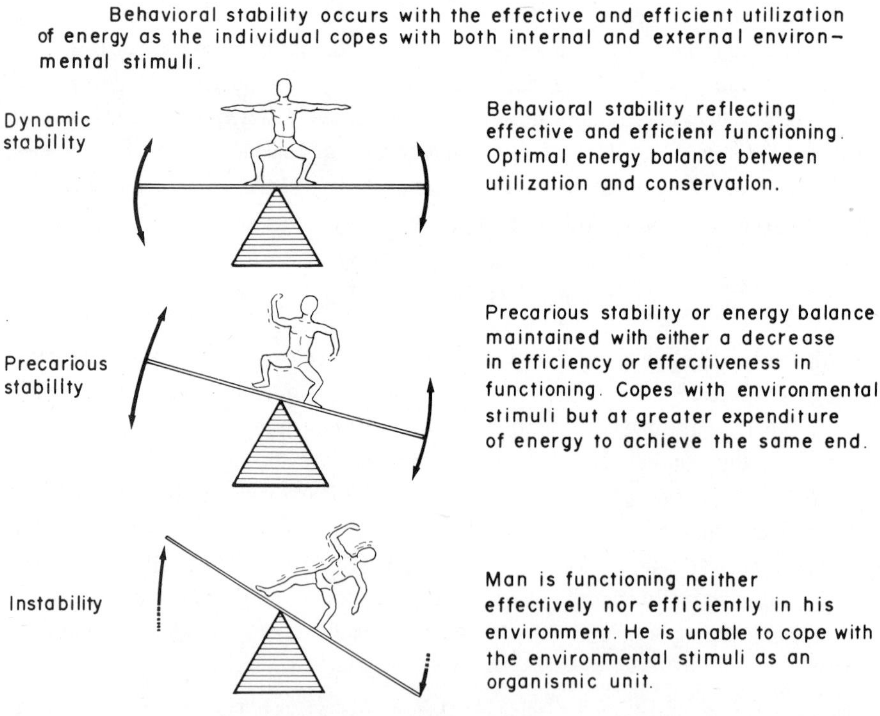

Behavioral stability occurs with the effective and efficient utilization of energy as the individual copes with both internal and external environmental stimuli.

Dynamic stability

Behavioral stability reflecting effective and efficient functioning. Optimal energy balance between utilization and conservation.

Precarious stability

Precarious stability or energy balance maintained with either a decrease in efficiency or effectiveness in functioning. Copes with environmental stimuli but at greater expenditure of energy to achieve the same end.

Instability

Man is functioning neither effectively nor efficiently in his environment. He is unable to cope with the environmental stimuli as an organismic unit.

Fig. 8. See-saw illustration of behavioral stability.

point. He keeps the board moving within controlled limits by gently shifting his weight from one foot to the other with the appearance of minimum effort. If he begins to lose his balance, the board swings in a wider arc and his body movements become quite exaggerated as he attempts to maintain control while regaining his balance. If he loses his balance completely, one end of the board hits the ground and he falls off.

The shifting position on the stability continuum can be demonstrated as a result of external environmental changes. Ordinarily, a person observed casually walking down the street utilizes movements that are both effective and efficient. Picture, if you will, that same person walking across a very icy street: he utilizes many odd body movements, with a corresponding increase in energy utilized in this activity as he attempts to maintain or regain his balance. His stability as a unified whole is very precarious. Should he be confronted by a skidding car bearing down on him, he probably would not be able to avoid injury. He would lose his balance and either fall getting out of the way or be hit by the car. In either event he moves to, or closer to, the point of instability.

Internal environmental changes can also cause the person's position on the stability continuum to be altered. A person who is drinking alcoholic beverages may be observed moving from a point of behavioral stability through precarious stability to a point of instability. After a few drinks, several inconsistent, incoherent, or disorderly behaviors may be identified. As the drinking progresses, his behaviors may become less efficient but still relatively effective. Eventually, a decrease is noted in both the effectiveness and efficiency of his behaviors. If the consumption is continued, the organismic behavior may become totally disorganized, inconsistent, and incoherent. Moving completely to the end of the continuum, the person eventually loses consciousness.

Recognition of precarious behavioral stability is the nurse's responsibility. Sometimes cues to a patient's discomfort, misconception about the disease, treatment, or role expectations are identified by noting an inconsistent, incoherent, or disorderly behavior. Something that the patient does or says is without logical connection, contradictory, or ill-timed; a few behaviors are generally lacking in agreement in relation to his other behaviors or the expected behaviors under the circumstances. These behavioral cues signify to the nurse that the patient is expending more than the usual amount of energy in his attempt to maintain or regain his steady state.

The average person tends to overlook incongruent behaviors both in himself and in others. Therefore, the student in nursing will need to compare and contrast his or her observations in the clinical setting with those of an experienced nurse for a period of time. With practice, the student will develop or refine these observational skills and become very adept at identifying the less obvious or covert behavioral cues. The statement that "all behavior has meaning" will become more significant when the observational skills are sharpened and the student has gained a solid theoretical base of knowledge about Man as a total functioning unit.

The nurse in the following situation utilized her observational skills and judgment to intervene to avert a potentially serious accident. A large, burly truckdriver was in line to receive a typhoid injection in a health department clinic. As he rolled up his sleeve in preparation for the injection, he commented to the nurse: "Shots don't bother me." The nurse, however, noted beads of perspiration on his forehead and a general muscle tautness. These behavioral features and actions were not in agreement with his words. As a precaution, the nurse unobtrusively seated the truckdriver in a nearby chair to receive his injection. As the needle touched his skin, the man fainted. The nurse's observation of his inconsistent and incongruent behavior and her foresight kept him from falling to the floor. Since he was already seated, he merely slumped forward in the chair for several seconds.

Although all people have a potential for energy imbalance and inappropriate allocation of their energy, it is more likely to occur when they become ill. When people become ill, the necessity for limitation or change in their usual activities may be frightening or threatening. They may find themselves in a situation where they have little knowledge and little to say about what is done to and for them. Their usual methods of organizing themselves within their environment must be altered and, consequently, their stability may become very precarious.

People differ in the manner in which they deal with the illness situation. It must be noted that the cooperative patient, as well as the one considered to be uncooperative, may have a precarious behavioral stability. The person who overtly exhibits an energy imbalance is frequently seen as "acting like a baby" or as exhibiting hostile, angry, or aggressive behaviors. However, the cues may be much more subtle in some individuals. The calm, friendly, cooperative facade often masks a frightened or insecure person. The nurse must carefully assess each individual to determine where he is on the stability continuum. This assessment will gain greater accuracy if there are data available regarding the patient's preillness behavioral patterns. What might be interpreted as an inconsistent, incoherent, or disorderly behavior may be one of his accustomed behaviors understandable in the context of his regular environment.

SUMMARY

The terms *care* and *comfort* may be interpreted by the patient and his family to mean energy-conserving measures that include having things done for him or "making it easier" for him. The nurse must help them to understand why this expectation is not always in his best interests. The goal of the nurse is to assist the patient with his adaptive processes so that within the limits of the illness situation, the patient will be functioning both as effectively and efficiently as possible and actualizing himself according to his nature. The nurse focuses on the stability of Man as a unified whole and the behaviors that indicate how he is apportioning his energy as he carries out his activities of daily living within the limitations of his illness situation. There are times when the steady state will only be regained if energy is expended; at other times it will be regained only if energy is conserved.

The degree to which the disease process and subsequent interferences with his accustomed activities of daily living are or may be disturbing to the person is determined by examining the individual's stability as an integrated behavioral unit. The nurse observes the consistency, coherency, and orderliness of the patient's behavioral features and actions in context with the norms for a similar population in a like situation. A judgment can then be made as to the patient's relative position on the stability continuum. The practitioner's expertise lies in his ability to assess the demands of a situation and to judge whether the patient is allocating his energies most productively. The nurse then encourages or assists the patient to increase or decrease his energy expenditure with a specific activity or set of activities.

There are several factors that always must be taken into consideration when assessing an individual's patterns of behavior and his energy allocation or behavioral stability. The next chapter will present a concept of structural variables that provides us with a systematic and comprehensive method of extracting, organizing, and evaluating the importance of generalizations that may be operative in a particular patient situation.

Chapter 4

STRUCTURAL VARIABLES
an assessment profile

Beginning nursing students often feel as if their feet are planted in midair because they view every patient situation as totally new and unique. They frequently find it difficult to accept the fact that patients are just ordinary people who are confronted with a foreign and frightening experience. Actually, however, students possess a wealth of information and life experiences that can assist them over this initial hurdle once they recognize that there are many more common denominators in the patient situation than they originally realized.

Throughout this book we have indicated that there are generalizations that can be made about Man as a species and about subgroups of the population; however, not all the generalizations hold true in a specific situation. There are several factors that provide a framework for determining which generalizations might govern the responses of a particular patient. This key set of factors will be treated as a concept and labeled *structural variables* and is introduced at this point to provide a method of examining those common denominators that enable a nurse to extract the most meaningful facts and theories in a particular patient situation.

DEFINITION

The concept of *structural variables* is defined as *those factors common to all men that will direct attention to the particular generalizations likely to be applicable to a specific individual.* The factors are considered structural because they give form to all interactions and structure every person's reactions in every situation. The factors are considered variables because they do not control or influence each person in the same way or to the same degree.

The factors common to all men are: (1) age, (2) sex, (3) religion, (4) ethnic or cultural group, (5) education and occupation, (6) relational: family group or significant others,* and (7) health status. Each factor represents a category or collection

---

*Usage of the term *significant others* is becoming more prevalent in nursing literature. People whom the patient considers most important in his interpersonal relationships may or may not be within his family or blood relative circle.

of generalizations that can be drawn upon to understand people who share the same or similar characteristics, traits, and beliefs. Although the exact nature of the factors varies from person to person, all the listed structural variables are applicable to every human being. For example, every person has a specific age; the relevant set of facts and theories will vary depending upon whether the person is 8, 18, or 80 years of age. Similarly, the generalizations about any specified religion vary just as widely as exemplified by Roman Catholic, Christian Scientist, Buddhist, Presbyterian, or agnostic beliefs.

A STRUCTURAL VARIABLE PROFILE

A composite of the factors listed above constitutes a structural variable profile for an individual. Thus every person has a profile that is comprised of his specific age, sex, the ethnic group or culture most dominant in his life, his primary and extended relational group that may consist of blood relatives or persons who have close familial type bonds, his dominant religious beliefs, the type and amount of his education and his occupation, and the status of his health. The nurse delineates a structural variable profile by identifying the specific characteristics of the factors for a particular patient. (See boxed material.)

While it is usually quite apparent that the individual's structural variable profile provides the context within which the needs of the patient are assessed, it is often less apparent to nurses that they, too, have a profile that is influencing the nurse-patient situation. You must recognize that as a person you also view the world, act, and in turn are reacted to through the network of your own structural variables.

STRUCTURAL VARIABLE PROFILES OF THREE INDIVIDUALS

Profile	Subject A	Subject B	Subject C
Age	22 years	67 years	9 years
Sex	Female	Male	Male
Religion	Catholic	Methodist	Protestant
Ethnic-cultural group	Philippino; U.S. resident 1 year	Unknown; born in Nebraska	Mexican-American
Education-occupation	R.N. with B.S.	Retired lawyer	Second-grade student
Relational	Lives alone, engaged, no relatives in U.S.	Widower living with son, son's wife, and two children	Lives with mother and five younger siblings
Health	Six months pregnant	Diabetes and prostatitis	Fractured left femur

(See Fig. 9.) Your own age, sex, familial background and experiences, cultural beliefs, religious tenets, educational level, and health status combine to influence your interaction with others. For instance, a middle-class health professional may find it very difficult to accept a decision by a ghetto dweller that he would prefer to remain at a lower level on the wellness continuum than he needs to because he will not "accept charity." On the other hand, a patient may have difficulty accepting health teaching from a nurse who is a member of a minority group or who is young enough to be a grandchild.

A two-step assessment process

For the evolving profile to become a useful tool for the nurse, the implications of the term structural variable must be fully understood. The use of this concept requires a two-step assessment process.

The first step is dictated by the word *structural*. We indicated on p. 40 that the

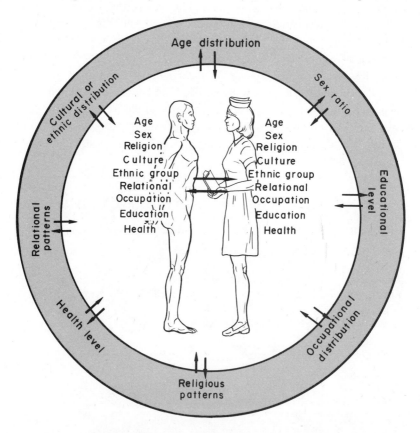

Fig. 9. Structural variables affect interaction between patient and nurse.

factors comprising the structural variable profile are considered structural because they give form to all interactions and govern every person's reaction in every situation. Therefore, the nurse must attempt to identify the generalizations that correspond with each of the factors indicated in a specific profile.

Although each person is unique, this is not a total uniqueness. Each person exists within a specific family, community, and society. Therefore, as a person is formulating his repertoire of regular and consistent behaviors, he will be influenced by the superordinate systems in which he exists as well as by the operation of the subsystems of which he is comprised. Natural and behavioral scientists have identified many commonalities among Man at the various behavioral levels.

There are several disciplines that have determined the behavioral norms for cellular, organ, and organ system functioning. For example, the age factor has been correlated with the maturation point of the body's temperature-regulating mechanisms and with the maturation of the nervous system to the point when voluntary bladder control is possible. Age and sex factors have been correlated with the usual expected subsystem behaviors and the corresponding organismic behaviors when considering the onset of menses as well as menopause. Sociologists and anthropologists have devoted themselves to identification of predictable behavioral responses of groups of people, families, communities, and societies. They have identified many major behavioral themes that help one to know and understand people of certain ages, races, and religions without knowing any one specific person.

The various disciplines have extracted the generalizations that typify the people under study, and you have very likely been exposed to many of these generalizations in high school or college courses. Thus, when you meet a person and identify his structural variable profile, you will have certain expectations of that individual's behavior. It is possible to anticipate many things that a person might be able or not able to do, might like or dislike, approve or disapprove, select or reject. One can anticipate some of the things that might be upsetting to the patient, things having the potential for disrupting his steady state as he engages in his ordinary activities of daily living while confronted with a stressor of a health-illness nature. *Thus the nurse is directed to identify all the generalizations that might be appropriate for an individual with a particular structural variable profile.*

The second or essential counterpart step is dictated by the word *variable*. We stated on p. 40 that these factors must be considered variables because they do not control, direct, or influence every person in the same way or to the same degree. Therefore the nurse is directed to determine the validity of the composite network of generalizations for the particular patient being assessed.

The connotation of the word generalization itself indicates that something is asserted to be true for all or *an indefinite part* of a particular class or membership.

Although many of the behaviors of an individual will reflect the major themes of the subsystems of which he is composed and the superordinate system in which he exists, each person will be tailoring his behavioral responses to meet his needs as he sees fit and as is genetically possible. For example, some children crawl, walk, and talk within the behavioral norm age expectations, and others do not. Some people adhere strictly to a particular set of religious beliefs in all aspects of their lives, while others may give only token acknowledgment to the tenets of their religion. *The nurse must determine the degree to which the generalizations actually hold true, the degree to which they actually govern or influence that specific patient's behavioral responses.*

Validation of cues

While the structural variables are integral factors that must be considered in assessing the needs of every individual, there is an inherent danger of which every nurse must be aware. This is the very common habit of stereotyping.

Stereotyping has three characteristics: (1) persons are categorized according to certain identifying attributes; (2) general agreement tends to exist on the attributes that persons in the category possess; and (3) a discrepancy exists between actual and attributed traits.

To categorize teenagers as resentful of authority and interested in fast cars, rock music, and smoking marijuana obviously is not an accurate assessment of many individual adolescents. Blacks have suffered particularly from the dangerous stereotype of being superstitious, lazy, happy-go-lucky, and ignorant.

All stereotyping, however, does not attribute unfavorable characteristics to the category. Boy Scouts are generally seen as wholesome, intellectually curious young men who help old ladies to cross busy streets or carry their bundles. Such a picture is shattered when one of this group is identified as a juvenile delinquent. The "American" image of the industrious, intelligent, ambitious, and progressive character is perhaps the most obvious example of attributing favorable attributes that are by no means shared by all members of the category.

Prejudice undoubtedly has a part in stereotyping. Certain racial or religious groups are assigned undesirable characteristics, while others are seen as totally favorable in spite of the fact that there are, without doubt, persons who do not fit the stereotype in each category.

It is essential that the nurse learn to utilize the structural variables as cues that must be tested in each individual case. One cannot assume that because a person has a Spanish surname, he will want only highly spiced food to eat. Not all men are stoic. Not all women are devoted mothers. Not all older persons are delighted to join the Golden Age Club to fill their lonely hours; in fact, not all older persons have an excessive number of lonely hours.

The danger of stereotyping can be minimized when nurses use the structural variable profile as a means to gather and organize the generalizations that might hold true in their patients' situations. Then the nurse can decide if these generalizations, in fact, do govern or direct the patient's behavior and, if so, the extent to which they do.

OVERVIEW OF STRUCTURAL VARIABLES

Having considered the importance of the structural variable profile in predicting possible behavioral responses of an individual, we will turn now to a brief discussion of each of these profile factors. This discussion is intended to indicate the usefulness of the factors for understanding and anticipating behavioral responses and in no way covers the full scope of each factor.

Age

The number of years an individual has lived is perhaps one of the most obvious structural variables in determining his behavioral responses at all levels. We know that a child will exhibit a markedly higher temperature elevation as the result of an infection than will an adult. Children have a higher metabolic rate than adults; thus, with the additional heat elimination necessitated by a fever, the temperature response is more marked. The elderly or very debilitated adult, on the other hand, may evidence little or no temperature elevation with infection. In either case, the nurse will consider the variable of age in assessing changes in temperature.

In caring for a bedfast patient, the age variable provides a particularly important cue. Most elderly individuals suffer from some measure of vascular degeneration; thus, turning and positioning may be more critical to prevent tissue ischemia than in a younger person whose vascular supply is more adequate.

The aged person who may have less adaptive energy than someone younger may also be less able to withstand a stressor than a younger person. The exertion of hoeing a garden, which most likely is good exercise for a man of 30, may be a stressor of major proportions for a man of 80.

In addition to physical reactions that differ with age, we must consider those differences in perception of a situation resulting from the individual's age. A child of 2 may be shamed by wetting his pants, but the effects of such shame are quite different for him than for a person of 48 who suffers from incontinence (loss of bladder control) as a result of a bladder infection.

The diagnosis of a fatal illness, on the other hand, may be less stressful for an aged person than for one who has reasonably expected many more years in which to achieve his life goals or who has dependents who will be left without a breadwinner in the family. The examples given here are only a few of the many that could be considered. Age can and does affect behavior at all levels of Man's organization.

There is an additional facet of the age variable that merits consideration. You are probably quite familiar with the developmental tasks of childhood. The child must be socialized to both primary and secondary groups, master verbal and written language, develop motor skills and manual dexterity, and learn those complex cultural patterns required for living as a self-sufficient adult.

Developmental tasks do not cease on reaching maturity, however. The young adult must learn to execute an occupational role in a satisfactory fashion. He usually chooses and learns to live with a mate and organizes and maintains a nuclear family. He may organize his life around some other meaningful primary group; however, in any case, he must assume responsibility for enforcing those social pressures that ensure continuity of his culture.

As individuals approach their later years, still more tasks must be carried out. A mother must find new ways to utilize her efforts once spent on rearing children. Older workers must relinquish responsibilities as they prepare to retire and must groom successors to provide continuity. New patterns of daily living and recreation must often be developed. Loss of friends and spouse often require major adjustments.*

Many of the developmental tasks, at any age, act as stressors in and of themselves. The energy required to accomplish the task can sometimes put the individual into precarious behavioral stability. Learning to adjust to retirement after a busy and productive career may precipitate some unexpected behaviors in a man.

Often the nurse will see a situation in which a patient's behavioral instability is far greater than would be reasonably predicted in the situation. For example, a woman whose left arm was broken in a fall evidenced unexpected precarious stability. Upon investigation, it was found that her youngest child had just enlisted in the army and she was having great difficulty working through her feelings of uselessness and loss. The additional stressor of the broken arm was simply one more factor to cope with at the same time she was attempting to deal with the stress of a developmental task.

Sex

Physiologically, the differences between the sexes are limited, but this structural variable is often an important influencing factor in an individual's behavior in a given situation. A female who is quite conscious of her physical appearance may have a totally different reaction to an ugly abdominal scar following an appendectomy than a male in the same situation. The acceptance of a therapeutic regimen that requires the patient to be in a totally dependent situation for all of his activities of daily living may, on the other hand, well be more acceptable to the female than to the male.

*For a review of developmental tasks, see Erikson, Erik H.: Childhood and society, New York, 1950, W. W. Norton & Co., Inc., especially Chapter 7, "Eight Stages of Man."

Societal expectations of acceptable male or female behaviors are well documented. In behavioral science courses you learned that the socialization process that every child goes through instills attitudes that make the socially dictated role acceptable to the individual. The "physically superior" male who will serve as breadwinner and protector of the female who will fill a subordinate role is still the norm, even though social change may be taking place to dispute this.

A man who had undergone back surgery was placed on complete bed rest and instructed that he was not to turn without assistance since correct alignment of his spine must be maintained. The nurse set up a schedule for changing his position every hour, but the patient became more and more uncooperative when she came in to turn him. After asking him several questions in an attempt to find out whether the procedure was painful or whether he understood why it was so essential that he turn regularly, he finally blurted out: "What kind of man would I be if I lie here and let a little woman hurt her back turning me over?"

This same structural variable has an influence on both the way a nurse perceives a given situation and is perceived by others in the same interaction. The female nurse must recognize that not only does she view a situation through a "female framework" but is seen by others within the limitations imposed by her sex. The patient mentioned before could not accept assistance requiring physical strength because he saw the nurse as too delicate for such activity. Male nurses may be rejected by female patients who find personal care by a male unacceptable, or a man may be very uncomfortable being bathed by an attractive young woman.

Religion

Religion, bearing as it does on such vital issues as the meaning and purpose of life, is often a powerful determinant in the individual's perception of and reaction to a situation. It is difficult for a patient to see himself as being cared for when tenets of his religion are being violated in that care. The Orthodox Jew may suffer great stress if the diet offered him violates the Laws of Kashruth.[1] The taboo against eating or preparing meat and milk together is often difficult to accommodate in a hospital diet kitchen since it requires totally separate dishes for preparation. The nurse who considers this structural variable can, however, alleviate this stressor for the patient by assisting the family in making arrangements to have food sent in from a kosher restaurant or in offering to heat and serve foods brought in from home.

The attitude of the young Catholic wife undergoing a hysterectomy may be quite different from that of a woman whose religion does not emphasize the role of procreation. By the same token, the attitude of a Catholic nurse toward a patient undergoing a voluntary abortion may serve as a stressor to the nurse.

Tenets of some religions can create a very real problem unless the nurse understands what underlies the behavior that is encountered. MacGregor[2] gives the example of the "uncooperative patient" from India who repeatedly violated orders for complete bed rest by standing gazing out of the window. It was found after some investigation that his Moslem religion dictated he look toward Mecca to pray five times daily. The simple expedient of moving his bed to a position from which he could face the prescribed direction for worship solved the problem and allowed him to cooperated with his therapeutic regimen.

While there is sometimes an overlap between ethnic origin and religion (the Italian is usually of the Catholic faith, the Greek of Greek Orthodox, and so on), this does not occur with sufficient consistency for us to consider them as one. In our mobile world society, religion has tended to become dispersed among various ethnic groups so that we must look at these variables as separate entities.

Ethnic or cultural group

Race appears to be more a social than a biologic phenomenon. Some ethnic groups have distinctive physical characteristics, but the physiologic makeup of all humans is the same. Moreover, all men have the same basic needs although the manner of meeting them may vary in some degree. There are some health deviations that appear more often within certain ethnic groups, but even this is often explained in terms of sociologic factors. The high incidence of diabetes among Jews is often explained to be the result of their tendency to marry others of their own Jewish background who also transmit this genetic disorder of metabolism. The higher death rate among black infants is related to poverty and the poor health care offered the large majority of this ethnic group rather than to physiologic differences.

The culture that develops within ethnic groups, however, is a powerful determinant in how a member of a given race reacts in a situation. Studies of individual's response to pain offer an example of the way in which different meanings may be ascribed to the same stimulus with resultant difference in reaction to the same stressor. Zabrowski's classic study compared the reaction of Jewish, Italian, and "Old American" genetic stock to pain. It was found that Jews and Italians tend to be quite emotional in their responses while the "Old Americans" reacted with stoicism, bearing pain with a minimum of outward expression.[3]

These culturally dictated responses to pain provide cues for the nurse who is assessing the patient's behavioral stability. A 40-year-old Jewish man hospitalized with abdominal pain was observed sitting up in bed clutching his sides and rocking from side to side as he crooned "Oi Yoi Yoi" repeatedly. The nurse initially viewed him as being in a state of very precarious stability but noted that when he was asked a question about subjects other than his pain, he relaxed visibly, dropped his hands to his lap, and conversed with no nonverbal indications of pain present.

Such reactions are a manifestation of the culturally dictated attitude toward behavioral patterns that are acceptable in a situation. Indeed, the stoic Jewish patient may be misunderstood and fail to receive the acceptance of his behavior by others of his cultural group. Much more familiar to us is the attitude toward the so-called "American" patient who fails to contain his emotional reaction in a similar situation.

Another factor that must be noted here is the cultural differences arising from place of residence within the United States. Differences in the incidence of certain disease conditions, life styles, food customs, and interactional patterns may be marked between the urban and rural population as well as between residents of the North, South, Midwest, West, or East. The aloof New Englander who communicates with few words is legend, as is the stereotype of the loud, aggressive Texan.

Regional differences, both imagined and real, become especially important when either the health worker or the patient is outside his own accustomed area. A patient from Georgia who was living in New York City was reported by a nurse to be very withdrawn and sullen at the outpatient clinic she attended for prenatal care. The public health nurse who made a follow-up home visit found that the woman had been laughed at several times in stores where she shopped because of her heavy southern drawl, and she had become reluctant to speak for fear of ridicule. She also expressed feelings of rejection since none of the neighbors in her apartment house had visited her home in the 3 months she had lived there. This perceived lack of acceptance as a person of worth was a major stressor to the individual who required help in adapting to a foreign area.

The health worker from the city may find it equally difficult to obtain acceptance in a rural area, where she is identified as an outsider. Such geographic factors must be identified as an integral part of the structural variables in such situations.

There exists a wide variation in the beliefs of what constitutes an acceptable level of wellness. In some cultural milieus, illness is seen as a punishment for misdeed or as a means to "prove oneself worthy" by acceptance of such a hardship. The criteria used by health workers may not be the same criteria used by a given cultural group. A department store clerk whose livelihood depended on standing on her feet for 8 hours a day consulted a nurse for advice because she had corns and calluses that made standing extremely painful. The suggestion that her problem could most likely be solved by consulting a podiatrist for minor surgery to correct the cramped position of her toes was met by indignant rejection. "What would people say if I had surgery just to keep my feet from hurting?" The cultural norms to which she conformed did not allow her to see this as a valid health need. She was willing to tolerate a lower level of wellness even with resources readily available to improve it.

We hear a good deal today about the "culture of poverty." While "the poor" can mean the black, the aged, the uneducated, or the sick, to name but a few, the subculture that encompasses this large group has rather distinct characteristics. Riessman and coauthors describe it as a culture whose long experience with power-lessness, hopelessness for improvement of their socioeconomic status, and lack of orientation to education has led them to a willingness to accept immediate gain rather than to postpone satisfaction. He characterizes them as present-oriented people who "have learned that it is futile to think of the future."

To work with persons from this group, the nurse must always be aware that her view of a desirable health goal may be quite different from theirs. A public health nurse working in a low-cost housing unit failed repeatedly to gain the cooperation of mothers in giving their babies the dry milk that was readily available to them. Her explanation that this would build strong bones and healthier children appeared to fall on deaf ears. When she changed her approach to the fact that the baby would sleep better and cry less if he received the milk, success was immediate.

This same present orientation provides an explanation for the difficulty often experienced in motivating such persons to bring their children into immunization clinics. These examples are, of course, generalizations but recognition that many people in such circumstances do share this type orientation to life increases the nurse's chance for success in gaining cooperation with a preventive health care program. As with all other structural variables, cues obtained from the individual's ethnic or cultural group must be checked out in the total situation for validation.

Education-occupation

The educational background and occupation of a person often appear to be two of the most obvious structural variables in evaluating the individual's behavior in a given situation. The nurse might well hypothesize that the blue-collar worker will be more willing to accept orders than a corporation executive. The explanation offered a patient with an elementary school education must often be quite different from that offered a college graduate. The complexity of explanations must be geared to the patient's ability to understand them.

While the basic needs of all individuals are the same, the establishment of need priority is often a manifestation of the environmental circumstances inherent in an occupational role. The physician who is hospitalized in his own small community may have great difficulty accepting the patient role under the care of personnel with whom he customarily interacts in a dominant role.

A waiter in an exclusive supper club developed emphysema and was advised to change jobs since the smoke-filled room in which he worked was aggravating his disease condition. After some consideration, it was his decision that he placed a higher priority on his above-average income than on his need for oxygen as long as he could possibly function in that capacity.

The occupational variable may also have a strong bearing on the degree to which certain behavioral pattern disruptions are disturbing to the individual. The traveling salesman whose eating patterns are often necessarily erratic because of irregular hours and accessibility of acceptable restaurants may be quite disturbed by a need for the carefully controlled diet of the diabetic patient. A debilitating chronic illness may be a greater threat to a manual worker than to a sedentary housewife. A loss of hearing may be more disturbing to a school teacher than to a production line worker or an accountant.

The correlation of this variable with income level provides many additional cues that must be tested out. Is the patient's income stopped abruptly when he is off the job? Is the secondary stressor of financial concern diverting energy needed in the cure process? Is it realistic to suggest that a person needs special low-sodium canned foods that are relatively expensive, or should less costly natural foods be recommended?

While education-occupation is an obvious variable, the reader is reminded that with this, as with any structural variable, the nurse must always be alert to the danger of stereotyping. To assume that every person who works as a manual day laborer has a limited ability for abstract thinking could be very inaccurate. To assume that a professor of English has good basic understanding of human physiology could be equally inaccurate. As with other structural variables, this factor must be considered in relationship to the total situation in assessing individual needs.

Relational

The role of the individual in relation to his own primary group is a structural variable that often exerts a strong influence on his behavior in a given situation. While we often think in terms of the nuclear, patriarchal family structure in this country, we must not assume this to be the relational variable for all individuals whose needs we are assessing. A matriarchal family structure, either acknowledged or not, is by no means rare, and the egalitarian marriage is becoming more common as more wives enter the job market. For some individuals a lifelong friend or a neighbor may be the "significant other." Increasingly, our society acknowledges the existence of family groups such as homosexual or communal relationships. The extended family pattern, while not common, is by no means nonexistent.

Whatever the basic structure of the person's relational affiliations, his role with his "significant others" has a direct bearing on his behavior in a situation. The extent to which a given stressor threatens his ability to maintain his family relationships may determine his pattern of adaptation. The entire family may be affected by one member's illness. If the father bears all the responsibility for family income, authority, and decision making, any event curtailing his function in these roles may disrupt all family functions. A mother's absence or incapacity may bankrupt family resources for its usual emotional support and affection. In the egalitarian family we find shared responsibility and thus often see a greater ability to adjust to the stressor of one member's illness.

One area to be considered in regard to the individual's relational variable is the number in the family. A family of ten obviously has more capacity for sharing responsibility than one of three. The person who lives alone and has only a neighbor to depend on has comparatively few resources available to him.

Perhaps one of the most critical factors in the family relationship to the nurse is the decision-making process it observes. When it is necessary or desirable to change certain behavioral patterns of an individual family member, the nurse must often determine which family member to work with to effect the necessary changes. A nurse who saw a German woman regularly in a doctor's office where she was under treatment for a skin disorder recognized after several weeks that the woman was not carrying out the prescribed orders for regular soaks and medication. When all efforts failed to change the woman's behavior pattern, the nurse hypothesized that the husband was probably the primary decision maker in the family and requested that he come into the office with his wife. After a discussion about his wife's condition, the regularity of her treatment improved and the condition was controlled.

These examples represent only a few of the situations and ways in which the relational variable affect the individual's behavioral patterns. The nurse will find this a vital structural variable to consider when assessing the needs of any patient or potential patient.

Health

In evaluating the effects of a stressor on an individual, the variable of health must always be considered. Is the person already expending adaptive energy to maintain behavioral stability in the face of another preexisting stressor? Has he sufficient resources to adapt without medical intervention? Just as the level of wellness that a person can attain and maintain is dependent on both genetic and environmental factors, so is his ability to deal with a given stressor.

Kogan suggests bluntly that: "All men are not created equal."[5] Indeed, every human being has his own unique genetic potential for health. A child born with a congenital anomaly may never be able to attain the same level of wellness as one blessed with superior physical integrity.

An individual's potential for health is also dependent on environmental factors. Does he have facilities for maintaining cleanliness and a nutritionally adequate diet? Or does he live in crowded conditions in which he is exposed repeatedly to communicable disease? Some jobs have inherent health hazards. Both the high-pressured coronary-provoking atmosphere in the corporation executive's office or the energy-consuming requirements made of the ditchdigger will have an effect on his ability to adapt to an additional stressor.

Three men suffered from carbon monoxide poisoning from a faulty heater in their place of employment. All appeared to be equally exposed. One of the victims overcame the effects of the poisoning and was released from the hospital in 2 days, but the other two responded very slowly. One, who had a chronic peptic ulcer, suffered from duodenal bleeding and required transfer to the hospital's intensive care unit. The other man had no obvious additional stressors but appeared to improve very slowly. Subsequent investigation revealed that 1 year earlier his wife had left him to marry another man, and since that time his behavior had been very erratic. He had been drinking heavily, often getting by on only a few hours' sleep, and eating a very inadequate diet. This situation represents three unique reactions to a similar stressor that could be explained only in terms of the individual's general level of health.

Utilization of the patient's health history can provide valuable information to the nurse as the patient's special needs are considered in the light of his structural variables.

OPERATIONALIZING THE CONCEPT OF STRUCTURAL VARIABLES

After considering a few, selected cues to be gained from each of the structural variables, let us consider now how the nurse can utilize this concept in planning and implementing care for an individual patient.

Mrs. Andretti, age 45, was admitted to the hospital with a diagnosis of cholecystitis and was scheduled for a cholecystectomy (removal of the gallbladder) in 2 days. She was suffering intermittent pain and was, as would be expected, in a state of precarious behavioral stability as she attempted to adapt to the multiple stressors in her internal and external environment.

In addition to the diagnostic tests and careful observation of cues to her level of behavioral stability that could be visualized at the organismic level, the nurse considered the possible cues to be gained from her structural variables. From information gained from her admission notes and a short conversation with her husband, the following profile and list of possible elements important to planning her care emerged:

1. **Age** At 45, she could be involved with the developmental task of accepting her children's independence of her.
   She could be menopausal.
   A surgical scar may not be a major concern to her.
2. **Sex** She will probably accept her enforced dependent role easily.

As a housewife, she will probably be the one to be instructed in preparation of the low-fat diet she will be required to follow when discharged.

She may be concerned about her appearance when she is in less pain.

3. **Religion** Ask if she wishes to talk to a Catholic priest before surgery.

Watch for a rosary on the bedside table or under the pillow so that it isn't thrown out with the linen or trash.

4. **Ethnic or cultural group** Italian ethnic origin supports the hypothesis of a matrarchal family structure.

She will probably display pain and fear quite overtly.

She may require assistance in monitoring the number of visitors so that she doesn't become overly tired.

5. **Education-occupation** She may be accustomed to talking with many people in a day since she clerks in the family grocery regularly.

Eighth-grade education may indicate a need to utilize less complex terminology and explanations to her.

6. **Relational** She may be uneasy about her four children even though the youngest is 17.

She appears to be the dominant decision maker in the family.

7. **Health** Overweight indicates need to encourage development of new eating habits.

History of frequent upper respiratory tract infections indicates special observation and care in turning, coughing, and deep breathing postoperatively.

By utilizing these hypotheses, the nurse was able to check out the cues provided by an analysis of Mrs. Andretti's structural variable profile and thus avoid many potential stressors at a time when her adaptive energy was needed to adapt to unavoidable stressors in her environment.

SUMMARY

The concept of structural variables provides the nurse with a method of identifying the generalizations likely to influence nursing interaction with the patient or potential patient and his family. Each time the nurse moves into a new situation, he or she will first determine the structural variable profile for all those involved. Once the profile has been identified, the nurse mentally selects and organizes the generalizations most likely to direct or influence the person's behavioral responses. Such analysis enables the nurse to identify a set of questions that must be answered and to develop a tentative working hypothesis before entering a patient situation. The nurse will continue to refine the initial hypothesis as he or she interacts with the patient, obtaining answers for questions and validating the original conclusions. By this method the nurse avoids the trap of prejudging and stereotyping of behavior. Thus, utilization of the concept of structural variables ensures that each person will be viewed as a unique individual by providing the nurse with a framework for identifying the most relevant questions to be raised, as well as bringing into focus the most appropriate facts and theories that help to understand and anticipate the particular patient's needs.

Attention must now be turned to a general philosophic examination of the concept of health, which will provide the background for the subsequent discussion of stress.

REFERENCES

1. Berkowitz, Philip, and Berkowitz, Nancy: The Jewish patient in the hospital, American Journal of Nursing **67:**2335-2337, 1967.
2. MacGregor, Frances Cooke: Uncooperative patients, American Journal of Nursing **67:**89-91, 1967.
3. Zabrowski, Mark: Cultural components in response to pain, Journal of Social Issues **8:**16-32, 1952.
4. Riessman, Frank, and others, editors: Mental health of the past, New York, 1964, The Macmillan Co.
5. Kogan, Benjamin A.: Health: man in a changing environment, New York, 1970, Harcourt Brace Jovanovich, Inc., p. 4.

ADDITIONAL READINGS

Brown, Esther Lucille: Newer dimensions of patient care: Part III: Patients as people, New York, 1964, Russell Sage Foundation, pp. 23-37.
Clark, Margaret, and Anderson, Barbara: Culture and aging, Springfield, Ill., 1967, Charles C Thomas, Publisher.
Goldsborough, Judith D.: On becoming nonjudgmental, American Journal of Nursing **70:**2340, 1970.
Jaco, E. Gartly, editor: Patients, physicians and illness, New York, 1958, The Free Press.
MacGregor, Frances Cooke: Social science in nursing, New York, 1960, Russell Sage Foundation.
McCabe, G. S.: Cultural influences on patient behavior, American Journal of Nursing **60:**1101, 1960.
Skipper, James K., and Leonard, Robert C.: Social interaction and patient care, Philadelphia, 1965, J. B. Lippincott Co.

Chapter 5

LEVELS OF WELLNESS
a continuum for assessment

Is a man who must take daily injections of insulin to control a diabetic condition
"well"?

Is a woman who has dysmenorrhea "sick"?

Is a man who has residual paralysis of his right extremities following a cerebral vascular
accident "sick" or "well"?

Is a boy who had an appendectomy 2 weeks ago "well"?

Is a woman who is pregnant "sick"?

Is a man who wears a cast for a broken arm "well"?

Is a man who has cerebral palsy "sick"?

Is a man who has an invisible friend who talks and listens to him "sick" when he carries
out his family and job responsibilities satisfactorily?

Is a person who has eczema "sick" or "well"?

The way in which one answers these questions depends upon the definition that
one has for "health." The confusion that arises when one defines health as "absence of disease" and attempts to dichotomize health into "sick" and "well" states
becomes very apparent as a group compares their answers to these questions. The
notion that a person is either "sick" or "well" has vague criteria and is too gross a
judgment to be used by the nurse. It is imperative that the health professional have
a workable concept of health to use as a tool in making observations and assessments of patients in order to determine a course of action.

BASIS FOR A DEFINITION OF HEALTH

There are three major elements that must be included in a definition of health to
make it workable for the nurse. The concept must incorporate the fact that health
is a dynamic, changing phenomenon and that Man is an integrated biopsychosocial
being. Last, but vitally important to the concept, health must be viewed on a
continuum and not dichotomized as a condition of one being either "sick" or
"healthy." The following discussion will reinforce the importance of including
these three factors in a concept of health.

Health: a constantly changing phenomenon

Most people have experienced a headache of a few hours' duration, indigestion following a meal, or a backache after sitting in one position too long. Many people have the flu or colds at intervals during the year and sometimes residual symptoms are present for several weeks. There are times when a person just doesn't feel as energetic or "up to par" as other times but continues with his usual routine without giving it much thought because he has learned that it is a transient situation. Since the steady state is maintained by effective and efficient activities of the regulatory processes at all behavioral levels, it should not be surprising that at intervals the demands may exceed the person's adaptive resources. Readjustments are continually being made so there are bound to be fluctuations in the level of wellness from time to time. Health, therefore, must be considered a constantly changing phenomenon. In the next chapter we will be examining the observable behaviors reflecting the activity of the automatic regulatory mechanisms and their relationship to the fluctuations in level of wellness.

Health: integration of biopsychosocial factors

Man as an organismic being is composed of a set of open systems, as discussed on p. 6. Therefore, a stressor* may be of a physical, psychologic, or social origin, but regardless of the origin, Man's response is that of a unified whole. The nurse must keep in mind that *all* these areas are affected in some way and the response that one observes is a result of *all* the adjustments occurring in all areas at any given time. Health is health and cannot be compartmentalized as "mental health," "physical health," or "social health." People do tend to look at segments of health, because there may be a greater dysfunction in one of the three areas that skews the overall symptomatic picture in one direction. For example, the symptoms of a salesman suffering with a bleeding peptic ulcer are indeed skewed toward consideration of his pressing physical needs, even though the physical manifestations of the ulcer could result from psychologic stressors such as worry about his declining sales volume or job security. This, in turn, could be triggered by social stressors, such as his need for additional income to stop his wife's nagging about "no money." The salesman's stomach symptoms could be the result of the totality of unsatisfactory economic and social adjustments to his life situation. We hasten to add that his symptoms could also have been the result of a purely physical stressor such as imbalance in production of glucocorticoids by the adrenal cortex. The physician's treatment may result in improvement of the ulcer condition, but at a later date maladaptive symptoms or composite adjustments may move in another direction if the actual stressor has not been identified and resolved. Another time,

---

*A stressor is any agent or factor causing a change.

the holistic response may be reflected by psychologic or social symptoms instead of physical manifestations of a bleeding ulcer. The composite adjustments to the same stressors, instead of being reflected by a bleeding ulcer, may be reflected by distortion of reality, psychotic behaviors, or divorce because of the disturbed social relationship.

The concept of Man as a series of open systems with a holistic response is well illustrated when the nurse sees a patient who is confused or disoriented because of a physical stressor such as an electrolyte imbalance. The nurse may also see a social stressor such as the initiation of divorce proceedings followed by a flare-up of one of the partners' rheumatoid arthritis condition. Consequently, it is essential that the nurse consider health as encompassing social, physical, and psychologic facets of Man simultaneously. The concept of health must incorporate Man as an integrated biopsychosocial being.

Health-illness—a continuum

Health is not an either-or situation. Seldom does a person's health degenerate or disintegrate instantaneously. There are usually clues of pending health problems with a gradually developing set of symptoms. Conversely, neither is health regained instantaneously. One is not sick at 8 A.M. and well at 9 A.M. Although this example is exaggerated, the point is valid. Many people make a distinction between sickness and wellness based upon their ability to "go to work." Hospital nurses too often fall into the trap of considering the patient sick until the hour of discharge and well when he leaves the hospital. Judgments of this nature ignore the transition period between "sickness" and "wellness" and tend to focus exclusively on the very gross problems.

Dichotomizing also ignores the fact that an individual may have a diagnosed pathologic condition such as multiple sclerosis, which affects muscle coordination, and yet be able to function in life as effectively as all other individuals of the same sex and age. Mrs. J. was a 31-year-old woman, married 10 years, who had multiple sclerosis and had been confined to a wheelchair for the preceding 5 years. Mrs. J. frequently said: "I'm not sick—my legs just won't work." She cooked, cleaned, and shopped from her wheelchair with some assistance from her husband. The community nurse viewed health on a continuum, so when Mrs. J. mentioned that she and her husband wanted a child very much, the nurse asked if they had ever discussed this subject with their doctor and was told that they had not. The nurse later contacted the doctor who said that Mrs. J. could have children but that it could be quite a difficult event. During the next home visit Mrs. J. again mentioned that she and her husband had been talking about her becoming pregnant, so the nurse encouraged them to visit the doctor to discuss the subject with him. As a result of both the nursing and medical intervention, the J.'s had a full-term baby girl. The child is now 6 years old and the J.'s have raised her without assistance, even though Mrs. J. has been confined to her wheelchair. Had Mrs. J. viewed herself as "sick" or been viewed as "sick" by the nurse, it is doubtful whether the J.'s would have ever had a child or the strong cohesive family unit that has developed.

The concept of health can best be viewed on a continuum. We would support the use of a "wellness" continuum as it emphasizes the constructive attributes or characteristics of an individual rather than the negative "what's wrong with him" disease conditions. The wellness continuum allows us to consider how successfully the individual is functioning *in spite of the health stressor,* whether it is sociologic, physiologic, or psychologic in nature.

The opposite or polar points on the wellness continuum are the "optimal" level of effective and efficient functioning at one extreme and "death," the ultimate of noneffective and nonefficient functioning at the other extreme. Health is a constantly changing phenomenon; therefore, it is necessary to consider a second dimension. The second dimension or axis is "time," with the two extreme points being birth and death. In Fig. 10 we have plotted the health status of two hypothetical individuals during their first year of life to illustrate how health can be viewed on a continuum. In this situation, Infant A was functioning at a higher level at birth than was Infant B. This difference becomes less marked as they grow and develop

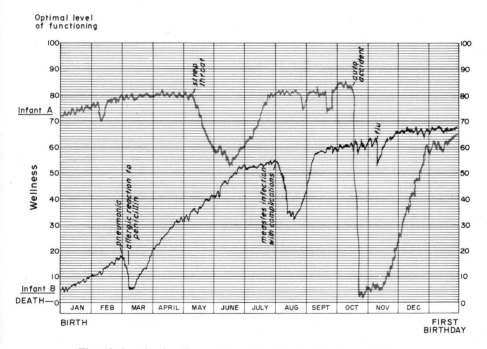

Fig. 10. Levels of wellness of two infants in their first year of life.

up to their ninth month, when the situation is suddenly reversed as Infant A came near death as the result of an automobile accident. As you study this graph, you will notice the small, daily fluctuations in the level of wellness and note the moderate to severe stressors that resulted in a lower level on the continuum for a temporary period.

A DEFINITION OF WELLNESS

A useful definition that incorporates the preceding ideas has been developed by Halbert Dunn. Dr. Dunn conceptualizes health on a *continuum* with wellness considered as a *dynamic* condition of change toward a higher potential of *integrated biopsychosocial functioning* within the ongoing and changing environment in which he lives. In Dr. Dunn's words:

High-level wellness for the individual is defined as an integrated method of functioning which is oriented toward maximizing the potential of which the individual is capable, within the environment where he is functioning.[1]

This definition of health correlates with the definition of the steady state presented on p. 9. A person who maximizes the potential of which he is capable within the environment where he is functioning will be seeking to actualize himself so that he will have a sense of accomplishment or fulfillment within the limitations of his situation.

The nurse who internalizes Dr. Dunn's definition will have a positive orientation toward health that creates a focus on the positive attributes and characteristics of the individual and the resources available to him in a given situation. This nurse will use herself as a catalytic agent to help people achieve an ever improving method of functioning within the limitations of their specific environments.

An integrated method of functioning

Again we emphasize that the stressor may be of a sociologic, physiologic, or psychologic nature, but Man's response is an organismic response representing his unified holistic attempt to cope with the stressor. The nurse will be oriented to the fact that the patient's response represents the sum of all the adjustments that are being made in an attempt to deal with the stressor. If a person is having a physical problem, it will affect how he views his world. His patience may be lessened or he may either avoid or seek more social interaction than he usually does. A person who is having difficulty adjusting to his job or to any other role may well have migraine headaches, "stomach" problems, diarrhea, or constipation. The increased tension may also manifest itself in frequent displays of temper, argumentative behavior, or silent, withdrawn behavior.

The nurse will recognize that if we were to see two patients of the same age, sex, religion, and cultural background, we could very likely see quite different responses at the organismic level. If two men had their right thumbs amputated, we might see one healing quickly and the man using the hand fully within 4 weeks. The other man might take much longer to heal, complain of severe pain, be troubled with phantom thumb sensations, and not use his right hand effectively for the rest of his life.

Because Man does respond as an integrated unit, one area may not be functioning within the "normal" parameters, yet other areas may well be compensating in such a way as to keep the overall level of wellness unchanged. A person may have a subclinical viral infection without knowing it because the body's defenses were able to cope with the invading organism. Of course, if the activity cannot be brought within the "normal" parameters, there will be an obvious change in level of wellness. There are times when the overall level of wellness remains unchanged even though the automatic physiologic mechanisms cannot correct a dysfunction. We might see this situation when an individual must utilize external aids such as phenobarbital to control a convulsive disorder or insulin to control a diabetic condition.

Maximizing the individual's potential

The question must be raised as to what extent or how well the individual is actually using his body or mind, which serve him as tools in his everyday life. The following examples illustrate two persons who are maximizing their potential. A 4-year-old boy was born without any arms. This youngster feeds himself with utensils held in his toes, buttons his clothing with his toes, and plays games with his six brothers and sisters. There is also a man who, as a result of an automobile accident, lost the use of both his arms and legs (quadraplegia). This man earns a living for himself and his wife by painting cards with a pen held in his teeth. He travels via wheelchair and car to shops, to church, and to friends' homes to socialize. In both examples the boy and the man are maximizing the potential of which they are capable. One was born with a handicap and the other acquired the handicap as a result of a car accident. Each was assessing the capacity that he had at his disposal and adjusting his behavioral patterns so that he was working toward achievement of realistically set goals.

The nurse must identify the positive attributes and characteristics of the patient and the degree to which he is capitalizing on them. This process involves assessing his adaptation or maladaptation as he attempts to cope with daily life in the presence of a health stressor. Assessment of the patient's potential functioning level is not carried out in isolation from the assessment by other health team members such as doctors, dietitians, physical therapists, or social workers. The nurse, when making the assessment, coorelates the medical diagnosis and treatment regimen established by the doctor, as well as information from other team members, with observation of the individual's functioning in daily life.

An individual may be terminally ill but have a relatively high level of wellness if he is adapting to the circumstances at his maximum level. This person is likely one who has come to terms with the inevitability of his own death and continues to maximize his remaining potential. He may need assistance with almost all of his physical functions, yet he functions as an integrated human being. He does not limit himself to a self-centered focus; he still sees himself as part of the world. He does what he can for himself based upon realistic expectations of his own performance. This person is utilizing his energies appropriately and his behavior is as effective and efficient as possible within his limitations.

The nurse may assess many positive attributes and characteristics of the patient that indicate that he is not maximizing the potential of which he is capable. There may be a wide discrepancy between the nurse's assessment of the patient's potential and his own evaluation of his situation. "Wholeness" or "worth" as perceived by the individual may be so distorted that his energies are expended nonproductively. This patient doesn't utilize capacities that remain available to him and, in a sense, the individual has given up "living." One occasionally hears of a group of people called "cardiac cripples." This term refers to those people who have survived a heart attack and have regained adequate heart muscle action yet continue to limit their physical activities unnecessarily even though the cardiac muscle will tolerate all their usual activity. These individuals have moved through the crisis and are so frightened of dying that they literally become vegetables. They withdraw from social activities, do not return to work, and undertake the very minimum of physical activity. These individuals, when viewed as a physical machine, may "get well" but as an integrated biopsychosocial being are achieving only a very low level of wellness. The nurse must recognize that her effectiveness will be hindered if the discrepancy between the nurse's and the patient's perception of his potential capacity cannot be reconciled.

Environmental factors affecting health potential

The nurse must assess the environment in which the patient is functioning in order to help him set realistic goals and capitalize on the positive environmental factors. Environment in this sense consists of all the influencing factors external to the individual. People, pets, furniture, sounds, odors, "tone" of the atmosphere, climate, and money available, to mention a few, are all potential influencing factors external to the individual. The characteristics of the significant others, such as educational level, religion, and age, would also be considered when assessing the environment in which the patient exists.

Some environments are conducive to a high level of wellness and others are not. A child with a physical disability has greater opportunity to learn to play with others if he has several siblings. The physical nature of the home itself will affect the degree to which the potential can be developed. For example, there was a patient living in a small mobile home who could not move from room to room because his wheelchair could not pass through the doorway unless folded, and he could not leave the trailer without assistance. These factors limited both the physical and mental stimuli available to him. Therefore, a change of residence was required before he could begin to maximize the potential of which he was capable. Some communities are more conducive to achievement of a high level of wellness than others because of the number and variety of resources available to its citizens. An Indian with a disability who lived on a reservation might have less chance to maximize his potential than if he lived in a metropolitan area that had such resources as rental equipment, home nursing services, physical therapists, dietitians, good public transportation systems, and educational programs for the home bound.

Each individual is unique and consequently the influencing environmental factors relevant to his particular situation must be identified. The nurse, patient, and involved "significant others" must identify and then attempt to take advantage of the positive environmental factors and to modify those not conducive to achievement of a high level of wellness.

ASSESSMENT OF LEVEL OF WELLNESS

No one has been able to define what an optimal level of wellness is for Man, nor have we a neat set of indices developed so that we can say that Mrs. Smith is at "X" position on the continuum of wellness. This is not a deterrent to a nurse, however, if the nurse seeks answers for the four questions inherent in Dr. Dunn's definition of wellness. The answers will give the nurse a specific direction for intervention geared to assisting the individual to attain an ever higher level of wellness. The inherent questions are:

1. What are the limitations with which the individual must cope?
2. To what degree is he utilizing the potential of which he is capable?
3. How does the individual view or evaluate his situation?
4. What are the environmental resources available to him? How can they be utilized more effectively?

Every one of us has potential for improving our functioning in daily life. In most instances, a person in a health crisis functions less effectively than usual, but hopefully only for a limited period of time. Hopefully, as a result of having successfully coped with the health crisis, the individual learns to function at a higher level than before the crisis. One goal of professional health workers is that each individual, either consciously or unconsciously, will apply knowledge gained through resolution of current crisis situations to resolution of similar health stressors or potential stressors in future situations. If this goal is achieved, the individual will cope more effectively and efficiently, thus maintaining a greater degree of behavioral stability. Ideally, the individual is constantly learning to adapt in ways that are conducive to the continual elevation of his level of wellness.

SUMMARY

Application of the concept of levels of wellness enables the nurse to assess the health status of an individual at the organismic level in a logical and definitive manner. The preceding questions reflect an attitude about the orientation to health that we believe enables the nurse to make a vitally important contribution to the patient's present and future well-being. In concluding, it must be added that the definition and orientation presented here is not unique to nursing. The very nature of the nurse's contribution as a health team member, however, makes incorporation of this perspective into daily practice mandatory if nurses are to maximize their unduplicated contribution as team members in the delivery of health care services.

REFERENCE

1. Dunn, Halbert L.: What high-level wellness means, Canadian Journal of Public Health **50:**447-457, 1959.

ADDITIONAL READINGS

Apple, Dorian: How laymen define illness, Journal of Health and Human Behavior **1**(3): 219-225, 1960.
Dunn, Halbert L.: High-level wellness for man and society, Journal of the National Medical Association **49:**225-235, 1957.
Dunn, Halbert L.: High-level wellness in the world today, Journal of the American Osteopathic Association **61:**978-987, 1962.
Freeman, Victor: Beyond the germ theory: human aspects of health and illness, Journal of Health and Human Behavior **1**(8):13, 1960.
Kaufman, Margaret A.: High-level wellness, a pertinent concept for the health professions, Mental Hygiene **47:**57-61, 1963.
King, Stanley H.: Perceptions of illness and medical practice, New York, 1962, Russell Sage Foundation.
Mechanic, David: Medical sociology, a selective view, New York, 1968, The Free Press.

Chapter 6

STRESS

common denominator of Man's responses to stressors

The fluctuations in level of wellness as discussed in Chapter 5 will be more clearly understood after a concept of stress has been explored. The stress concept will also provide a unifying thread for understanding Man as an integrated behavioral unit who is coping with new, different, or threatening changes in his daily life. Nurses have the responsibility for helping the patient to modify his daily living behavioral patterns in a manner that supports the physiologic processes necessary to regain or maintain stability. Therefore, the nurse must be able to utilize generalizations about the stress state and the underlying physiochemical regulatory behaviors that come into play when the steady state is threatened. An understanding of the stress state will provide a basis from which to begin working with patients who have a wide variety of clinical diagnoses.*

This chapter will be presented in three major segments. The first section will develop a concept of stress and examine its relationship to the steady state. The second section contains a brief review of the two subsystems most responsible for the physiologic changes observable when the stress state intensifies. The final section operationalizes the stress concept with a nursing assessment tool that focuses the nurse's observations on Man's responses as a unified whole.

A CONCEPT OF STRESS

The term *stress* is a simple and familiar word used frequently and understood by everyone when it is used in a very general context. The term, however, is understood by very few when an operational definition is desired that is sufficiently specific to enable precise usage in a clinical sense. A student who goes to the literature will find ''stress'' defined in many ways, and these definitions vary greatly in their point of emphasis.[1-6] Frequently, in nursing, confusion arises because the term is used interchangeably to mean either a cause or an effect. We therefore have found it

---

*This common denominator approach lays the foundation for subsequent examination of specific clinical entities, the depth and scope of which will be determined by the type of nurse or level of preparation to be achieved.

necessary to provide a definition that on the conceptual side enables nurses to integrate facts and theories from related sciences such as physiology, psychology, sociology, and medicine and that on the practical side offers a route for understanding the problems that the nurse will be encountering in her contacts with patients and potential patients.

The term *stress* will refer to *a state that is always present in Man but that is intensified when there is a change or threat with which the individual must cope*. The term *stressor** will refer to *the factor or agent that causes an intensification of the stress state*.

The steady state was defined in Chapter 1 as that state existing when energy is allocated in such a way that Man is freed to actualize himself according to his nature, maintained by effective and efficient activities of the regulatory processes at all behavioral levels, coping with the ever changing internal and external environments. Kahn and others point out that the steady state for Man, unlike machines, is not a "zero load" condition.[7] Rather, it is a condition of load roughly balanced with capability. McGrath indicates, as an assumption, that Man has an inherent need to use existing capabilities and that lack of opportunity to use his capabilities leads to atrophy or other malfunction.[6] Thus, when either an overload or an underload imbalance occurs, the stress state will likely exceed the limits of the steady state.† Before continuing with the examination of the relationship between the stress state and the steady state, there are several points about stress that must be made in order to provide a firmer foundation for such analysis.

Stress: an intangible abstraction

Stress, as a state, is an intangible abstraction that cannot be observed directly. Stress can only be recognized indirectly and its intensity measured by observation of symptoms or manifestations. Air movement is also an intangible state that is measured indirectly. This similarity allows air movement to be used as an analogy to illustrate that even though stress itself is an intangible item, its presence and intensity can be measured by indirect indices. The state of air movement is the result of differential changes in atmospheric pressure (the stressor). Air movement is not directly visible, yet there are characteristic signs and symptoms that usually enable us to recognize and measure its intensity. The degree of tree limb movement, the amount of dust blowing, and the pressure felt as one is walking down the street are but a few of the measurable items often used to determine the presence and intensity of wind. When these manifestations are absent, we customarily speak of "no wind." In actuality, we are referring to the fact that differential pressure changes are so slight

---

*Term coined by Dr. Selye.[1]

† More advanced courses will consider the overload and underload conditions in relation to such problems as sensory disturbances and social isolation, to name but two.

that we cannot identify any signs or symptoms of air movement. Just as with air movement, stress is always present although the changes may be barely perceptible when Man as a unified whole allocates his energies so that there is a balance between conservation and utilization of his energies. We can only surmise the presence of stress by identifying signs and symptoms at the observable organismic level or, in some cases, at other levels through the use of diagnostic techniques or instruments such as blood tests, x-rays, or thermometers.

Stress: necessary for life

Without a state of stress a person would cease "to be." Stress is essential both for the existence of life and of growth, since the human organism's viability depends upon constant mediation between environmental demands and his adaptive capacities. The various automatic self-regulatory mechanisms are in constant operation, adjusting to the continually changing nature and number of the internal and the external stressors. There are few surface or directly observable symptoms because the majority of these activities takes place within specific parameters or limits. Only when the activity intensifies and the limits of the steady state are exceeded do we become aware of the stress state. The average person ordinarily equates the term *stress* with a negative, uncomfortable, or frightening feeling. However, as defined in this chapter, stress is always present and, in moderation, the state can serve constructive purposes for Man, while an extremely intense state can lead to exhaustion and death.

The stress state is intensified when there is either a change in the rate of a given activity or when there is an alteration in the variety of behaviors required as the person is attempting to adjust to the stressors. The process of coping, which is often accompanied by an intensified stress state, is an essential ingredient for life. There are times, however, when the magnitude of the stress state is not in proportion to that required to cope with the stressor. For instance, a person who is faced with new, different, or threatening stressors may not be aware of the exact rate or variety of activities necessary for him to cope with a stressor while continuing to maintain a steady state. A person may undertake more activities than usual in order to avoid thinking about his problem situation, or he may focus on it to the exclusion of other daily activities. An individual may run when walking would suffice, or he may lower his voice when he needs to shout. In other words, either a greater range and rate of activity will occur than is necessary, or the situation may be underestimated and an insufficient rate and number of required behaviors will be used. It is during this period that the individual may have feelings of great discomfort until the stressor is resolved.

Fortunately, each time the individual is exposed to a stressor he tends to learn the nature and degree of activity required to resolve the situation and he develops greater facility for handling the demands with which he is faced. For instance, muscles develop greater capacity by usage, and the antibody system becomes more efficient in a crisis when there has been previous exposure to the same or similar microorganisms. Additionally, an individual's ability to cope with multiple stressors simultaneously is developed by frequent but milder situations where he has been bombarded by several stimuli at once. The individual becomes less vulnerable to the stressor, or like stressors, and is less apt to exceed the limits of the steady state when adjustments are called for. Consequently, intensification of the stress state can be a positive factor in the process of living.

Stress: phases of the intensification process

Actually, when intensification of the stress state occurs, the underlying activity can be viewed in three phases: alarm, resistance, and exhaustion.[8] Knowledge of these phases is helpful to the nurse who is assessing the individual's potential energy allocation in order to determine supportive measures for the patient whose behavioral stability is in question. These phases provide a basis for anticipating times when a patient may be more vulnerable to stressors. Moreover, understanding of these phases will support our preceding discussion of the constructive consequences of stress.

The phases of the stress intensification process are the same whether considering a very localized threat such as a broken toe or a generalized threat such as a severe systemic infection or pending surgery. However, the nature and number of regulatory behaviors involved will vary depending upon whether the localized responses can correct the problem or whether total body responses are needed. In the course of human life, everyone goes through the alarm and resistance phases an infinite number of times and into the exhaustion phase occasionally. Reversal of these phases can occur at any point as long as the individual's adaptive resources have not been entirely exhausted.

The *alarm phase* is the *short trigger phase* when Man, consciously or unconsciously, perceives a stressor and prepares to act. The very initiation of the alarm phase is useful since it sets in motion the mental and physical mechanisms that prepare Man for fight or flight. The nurse can capitalize on the purpose served by the alarm phase by developing an ability to make clinical judgments regarding the nature and timing of the forewarning an individual is likely to need in order to mobilize his adaptive behaviors most appropriately. If the nurse knows that a patient is going to be exposed to a new stressor such as a lumbar puncture for diagnostic purposes, shortly before the procedure she might inform him of what will occur and the expectations for his behavior. In this way, the nurses can assist the patient to move through the alarm phase and into the second phase of the stress intensification process so that he can better tolerate the procedure.

Since the alarm phase is just a short trigger phase, however, the nurse knows that if information is given too far in advance, the alarm phase is initiated but a reversal will automatically occur if the stressor does not materialize. Therefore, the patient will be just as vulnerable as before or may even be in a more vulnerable position. This increased vulnerability can be demonstrated by the woman who is pregnant for the first time and repeatedly confuses false labor with true labor. With the onset of some contractions, the woman follows a carefully planned course of action. However, when she arrives at the hospital, she is examined and told to return home since she is having false labor. She does so and awaits contractions that are closer together and more rhythmic. A few days later she returns to the hospital only to be told the same thing and to be given the same instructions. She is now in an even more vulnerable position because she is absolutely determined not to be alarmed again by false labor. Consequently, she ignores the true warning signals and allows the real labor processes to proceed too far before initiating action. She becomes extremely frightened and is finally rushed frantically to the hospital by her husband. She may make it into the delivery room, or she may deliver the baby in the car unattended. Her expected adaptive responses did not occur because the true stressor had not materialized as anticipated on the first trips to the hospital, and thus she was unprepared when it did occur.

There are other times when the nurse will decide to give no forewarning of a pending stressor. Some patients, during the waiting interval, will imagine all sorts of things or become emotionally upset. They may exhaust their adaptive resources before the procedure is undertaken. The nursing intervention will be based on an assessment of the patient's behavioral stability and his adaptive capacity, as well as the nature of the stressor.

The second or *resistance phase of the stress intensification process is where adaptation hopefully occurs.* The body's physiologic forces are mobilized to cope with the stressor; however, resolution of the stressor may entail modification of the external as well as the internal environment. Therefore, some alteration of the person's customary deliberative behaviors usually accompanies the subsystem changes in the resistance phase.

As indicated earlier, this stage can have long-range value as well as immediate positive consequences for an individual. Each time the individual mobilizes his defenses successfully he is, in effect, learning how to cope effectively and efficiently with the stressor. For the college freshman, the testing procedure is a very real stressor that can cause an extremely intense stress state. As the student becomes test wise and develops good study habits, stress will probably be less intense before subsequent examinations.

The *third phase is that of exhaustion.* This is the phase where the positive results of regulatory behaviors are diminished and death can be the ultimate consequence.

The exhaustion phase represents the period when the person's adaptive energy resources have been overtaxed; he is no longer able to deal with the threats or demands placed on him. Unless new stores of adaptive energy can be mustered, death will inevitably follow. Although reversal can occur in this phase, it often requires external resources to provide additional adaptive capacity. Blood transfusion, massive dosage of antibiotics, or institutionalization for psychotherapy and chemotherapy are examples of measures that might be utilized in an attempt to reverse the process.

MARGIN OF SAFETY

With the preceding background comments about stress in mind, we are now prepared to examine the nature of the relationship that exists between the stress and the steady states.

If the stress state consistently or drastically exceeds the limits of the steady state, the results may become less constructive or actually hazardous for the individual. To clarify this statement, we will go one step further and suggest that there are actually two sets of limits to be considered. The survival or outer limits are those limits that cannot be exceeded if life is to continue. The steady state is demarcated by an inner set of limits, within which Man has an internal constancy and is in harmony with the environment in which he exists.

The difference or area between these two sets of parameters constitutes a safety margin for behavioral responses. When the behavioral responses are outside the limits of the steady state, there will be a fluctuation in a person's level of wellness. We view this gray area positively since signals of the need for corrective action become apparent. Often, the individual himself will recognize this fact and will institute the essential corrective activity, but sometimes he will require assistance. In other words, the individual has a margin of safety where action can occur before the situation becomes irreversible. These notions can be visualized in Fig. 11.

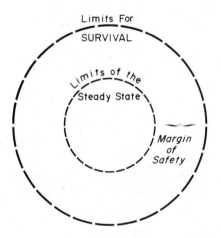

Fig. 11. Man's margin of safety between the limits of the steady state and the limits for survival.

It must be recognized that the parameters constituting the steady state will not necessarily be the same for any two people, since the amount of energy available is genetically determined. Each person develops his potential for coping with stressors to a different degree.* Moreover, it appears that some people have a greater quantity of readily accessible energy than others; consequently, some persons may have a wider range in the steady state than others have.

Students often ask the very reasonable question: "What are the parameters for the steady state and for survival?" The most honest answer is: "We don't know." This answer does not make the general concept any less useful. It is similar to the answer that would be given if the question were: "What are the parameters of the color orange?" All of us can identify the color orange, but on the color spectrum who can say exactly where orange begins and ends? We know something about the specific physiologic conditions† contributing to the overall steady state and have some knowledge about some of the survival limits, but this knowledge is isolated and limited. Hopefully, as modern science advances and research techniques and methodology are improved, this question can be answered with greater specificity.

If Man's regulatory behaviors are overtaxed and the limits of the steady state are exceeded, there will be identifiable behavioral cues at the organismic level. In Chapter 3 the notion of a behavioral stability continuum was presented. That continuum can now be superimposed upon Fig. 11 in such a way as to demonstrate the correlation of the organismic behavioral continuum with the steady state and the limits of survival. (See Fig. 12.)

---

*Note hypothesis about energy in Chapter 1, p. 0.
†Conditions such as body temperature, blood pressure, acid-base balance, and the like.

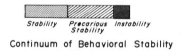

Stability   Precarious   Instability
Stability

Continuum of Behavioral Stability

Fig. 12. Correlation of concept of behavioral stability continuum with the steady state and survival limits.

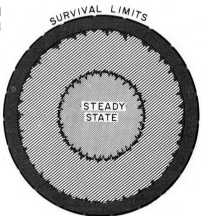

The nearer the behavioral responses are to the red area in the diagram, the greater is the danger of instability or actual threat to survival. Obviously, when behavioral responses are closer to the outer parameters that constitute the survival perimeter, the individual is much more likely to require assistance to cope with his problems. If the individual's behavior constitutes a threat to other people, intervention may be initiated whether he desires it or not.

Nurses must become adept at recognizing the signs and symptoms of intensified stress in their patients. Additionally, nurses must develop the ability to identify potential stressors that the patient may encounter and anticipate the intensification of stress that might result. Judgment must be developed in order to determine when nursing actions should be initiated to alter the stressor and when the most appropriate action is to support the patient's own adaptive mechanisms as he deals with the stressor. In many cases, of course, the latter may be the only option available, although the nurse is often in a position to modify situations that may be acting as stressors to the patient. Disruption in behavioral patterning (discussed in Chapter 2) is an area of potential distress that is often within the realm of the nursing staff to prevent or correct.

Stress: an indivisible state

Man, as previously defined, is a biopsychosocial being who responds as a unified whole. A given stressor may be categorized as a psychologic or social or biologic stressor, but we can speak of only one total state. Although the terms *psychologic stress* and *physiologic stress* are sometimes used, this is an artificial division of the stress state used primarily to make presentation of some subject matter more manageable. It is our firm conviction that nursing assessment and intervention will be hindered unless the nurse accepts the constant interplay among the various systems and considers the resultant state from the holistic perspective. Nursing intervention will be less than effective if nurses divide stress into different entities such as psychologic stress and biologic stress when the resultant state is, in fact, singular, and the patient can only be observed and treated as a unified whole.

VARIABLES ALTERING THE STRESS STATE

In order to anticipate or predict more accurately the behaviors that will occur in response to a stressor, it is necessary to consider the variables altering an individual's responses to a stimulus. Many people tend to think that there is always a direct correlation between the intensity of the stressor and the coping behaviors used to maintain stability. Although this may be true in many instances, often the protective or adaptive behaviors utilized may be either excessive or insufficient to cope with the stimuli. When making an assessment, the nurse must consider all of the following interrelated variables in context with the individual's structural variable profile:

1. Nature of the stressor
2. Number of stressors to be coped with simultaneously
3. Duration of exposure to the stressor
4. Past experiences with a comparable stressor

Nature of the stressor

Different kinds of stressors will cause varying degrees of activity. An interesting example of this involved a patient who had been having daily vitamin B_{12} injections. He informed the nurse one night that he was having difficulty sleeping, but when the nurse walked in with a sleeping pill for him, he refused to take this medication. He became very upset; both his pulse and respiratory rates increased, and in a higher pitched voice he told the nurse of his fear of becoming a "narcotic addict." In this case, the injection of a vitamin medication did not cause an intensification of the stress state, but the thought of a habit-forming sleeping pill did.

The magnitude of the stressor will also cause varying degrees of activity. The behaviors utilized to cope with a first-degree thumb burn or death of a classmate usually enables the individual to reestablish a steady state with a minimum increase in energy utilization. However, if the stressor's intensity is increased such that the individual suffers third-degree burns over 90% of his body, or if he is faced with the death of a spouse, the coping behaviors may not be adequate to reestablish the steady state, and death can occur as a result of either stressor.

Number of stressors to be coped with simultaneously

A person may cope successfully with a number of stressors at one time. However, there comes a point where stressors' demands for energy utilization exceed the resources available. If the individual has not established appropriate priorities for energy allocation, his behavioral stability will decline, and he will move to a precarious or unstable position on the stability continuum. A mother who returns home from the hospital following a hysterectomy and immediately attempts to resume all of her usual activities such as child care, cooking, cleaning, bookkeeping, washing, and ironing may dissolve into tears when her husband calls to say that he has to be out of town on business for a few days. Ordinarily, she has coped with her husband's absence in a matter-of-fact way, but in this instance she is unable to since she doesn't have the energy resources left to deal with the added responsibilities.

The reader should also recognize that in the preceding case the woman and her husband are dichotomizing between health and illness and therefore are ignoring the fact that she hasn't yet regained her usual level of wellness. She is not allocating her energies appropriately; she resumed her usual activity priorities without recognition of the energy required for completion of the cure process. Her husband's expectations for her performance were also unrealistic. Their orientation to health as the absence of disease is an additional stressor that contributed to the woman's precarious behavioral stability.

A more vivid example of multiple stressors concerned a woman whose doctor informed her on a routine physical exam visit that she had a lump in her breast that would have to be biopsied. She was scheduled for surgery 3 days later and told that in his opinion they would find a fatty cyst that could be removed without difficulty. Two days later the doctor was notified that his patient had committed suicide. The office nurse said that they just couldn't believe it because the woman had given evidence of stability during her discussion with them. They did not know that on the day she learned of the breast lump she arrived home to find that her husband had moved out. The next morning this woman was informed that her only son had been killed in an automobile accident. Any one of the three stressors—potential for disfigurement, loss of a husband, and death of an only child—would severely tax any individual's adaptive resources. The cumulative effect of the three was too much for this woman, and she gave up living.

The preceding examples demonstrate that when an individual is expending more than the usual amount of energy in order to maintain effective and efficient behaviors, the addition of one more stressor may lead to various degrees of disorganization of behavioral responses. It is helpful to remember this fact in a situation where a person may appear to be over- or underreacting to a particular stimulus or stressor.

The effect of the intensified stress state itself cannot be ignored. The more intensified the stress state, the more likely the state itself is to become an additional stressor to the person. The nurse must recognize that there is an inherent self-perpetuating element in the process itself that must be dealt with. When the stress state intensifies, the individual often becomes more vulnerable to additional stressors, and if he is unable to allocate his energies appropriately, there is a great risk that the state itself will become a stressor.

A familiar example of this situation is the student about to take final examinations. Whether his stress state will exceed the limits of the steady state depends upon his ability to allocate his energies appropriately and to institute effective and efficient behaviors. If he worries about the examination and doesn't allocate his energies productively, his ability to concentrate and retain what he is studying will be diminished. When the stress state exceeds the limits of the steady state, it may become an additional stressor so that in an attempt to compensate for his decreased ability to study effectively, the student may study many more hours. Consequently, he may get less sleep than usual (a stressor) and may eat more irregularly (a stressor), which causes additional intensification of the stress state, and his anxiety may cause him to perform poorly on the examination.

Another student in a similar pretest situation may be unable to take the examination because of a severe respiratory infection. Under ordinary circumstances, his physiologic coping behaviors probably would be sufficient to control the invading organisms without disruption of his overall behavioral stability. However, the intensified stress state (commonly labeled anxiety in this case) has become a stressor, making him more vulnerable to the circulating microorganisms because his adaptive capacities have been severely overtaxed. Usually, the intensification process can be reversed when the student is confined to his bed, which creates a climate for constructive reallocation of his energies and restoration of the steady state.

We can conclude that an individual's vulnerability at any given time can be related to the number of stressors he is faced with simultaneously. The nurse recognizes that what may be considered a relatively insignificant stressor in one set of circumstances may be very significant in another. It must also be remembered that the intensified stress state itself can become a stressor to the individual, in some instances.

Duration of exposure to the stressor

Continued exposure to a stressor can exhaust a person's adaptive resources. It is helpful to look at Man's general resistance level as presented by Dr. Hans Selye.[1] He indicates that in the acute phase of the alarm reaction the general resistance to the particular stressor falls below normal. Then, as the individual responds with the activation of his adaptive processes, the capacity to resist rises considerably above normal. However, more than the usual amount of energy is required to sustain these adjustment activities. Eventually, in the exhaustion phase, resistance again drops below normal as his energy resources become depleted. (See Fig. 13.) Man can

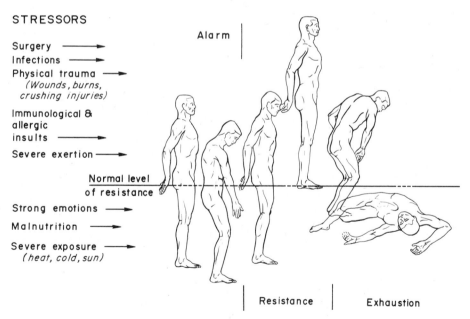

Fig. 13. Phases of the stress intensification process.

only sustain his adaptive processes above his normal level of resistance for a limited period of time. If the exposure is continued, eventually his energy reserves are not sufficient to meet the demands of the situation, and he will enter the exhaustion phase, where he can no longer maintain effective and efficient behaviors. In other words, continued exposure to one unresolved stressor, or one stressor superimposed upon another, reduces a person's ability to resist their detrimental effect as time elapses.

Past experience with a comparable stressor

If a person has not had previous experience with a stressor, his responses may be inappropriate. A person who has never eaten authentic Mexican food and innocently adds a liberal portion of spicy hot sauce to his enchiladas will probably experience a painful burning sensation in his throat and mouth and tingling of his lips. This individual usually reaches for the water glass, which will simply accentuate his misery, instead of the bread or tortillas that can alleviate it. However, if the person adds just a little bit of the hot sauce and eats some bread when he experiences a burning sensation, he may gradually develop a liking for the Mexican food.

If a person has had past experiences with a stressor, these experiences may predetermine the nature of his responses to a like stressor in either a negative or positive direction. For example, experience with a previous pregnancy may predetermine a woman's response to subsequent pregnancies. One woman who had suffered with rheumatoid arthritis for 10 years discovered that she was pregnant for the fifth time and was delighted. Although the deformities remained, the only time this woman had been free of joint discomfort during the past 10 years was when she was pregnant. (The normal hormonal changes occurring during pregnancy had caused a remission of her symptoms.) Another woman who discovered that she was pregnant again became extremely upset because she had had "7 months of misery" with both previous pregnancies.

Sometimes past experiences are unexpected stressors that the nurse must identify and cope with. A mother agreed to take her 5 year old to the county hospital outpatient clinic for follow-up of a possible hearing defect after consultation with the school nurse. When she failed to appear for three successive appointments, the nurse made a home visit to reassess the situation. The nurse finally discovered that 6 years previously the mother had had a terrifying experience while driving across a high suspension bridge, and she was still unable to drive an automobile across any bridge. Even when riding as a passenger in a car crossing a bridge, she had a very intensified stress state. She reported her symptoms as ashen color, cold extremities, diaphoresis (perspiration), increased respiratory and pulse rates, and a "bowel that feels like lead." The county hospital was located across the river from the family's home, and rather than tell the nurse about her problem, the mother had just failed to keep the appointments.

When considering past experiences, the nurse always keeps in mind that no two people will respond exactly alike when exposed to the same stressor, nor will the same person necessarily respond in the same way to the same stimuli at different times. The nurse will attempt to determine whether the stressor will evoke positive or negative effects and will attempt to determine the degree of intensification that may occur or is occurring.

Now that a concept of stress has been presented, we are ready to review the subsystem activity reflected in the totality of Man's response to a stressor.

BEHAVIORAL CLUES REFLECTING UNDERLYING PHYSIOLOGIC CHANGES

When the stress state intensifies, there are observable behavioral manifestations reflecting the underlying automatic cellular, organ, and organ-system behaviors. There are usually clusters of responses that occur together when the limits of the steady state are exceeded. These behavioral clues are useful in judging the intensity of the stress state. Although there are many structures within the body involved in maintenance of internal constancy, we will focus on the two systems responsible for most of the observable behavioral changes when the stress state intensifies.

The endocrine system and the autonomic nervous system are responsible for control, coordination, and integration of many of the physiologic regulatory behaviors. Both of these systems are influenced by stimuli from feedback mechanisms within the systems themselves as well as input from other systems within the body. Additionally, both systems are influenced by Man's emotions; both a person's feelings and thoughts can trigger changes within the internal milieu. This latter fact has many implications for nursing intervention that we will examine later on.

Endocrine system

The endocrine system controls the rate of tissue growth, cellular metabolism, fluid and electrolyte balance, and reproduction. The system is responsible for regulation of certain cellular processes in such a way that internal constancy is maintained. When the stress state intensifies, the endocrine system alters metabolism, circulation, and fluid and electrolyte balance to create a temporary internal environment that will sustain the life processes.

A localized stressor is managed by a local inflammatory response without evoking the adaptive processes of the endocrine system unless those local responses are not successful in dealing with the stressor. A sliver in one's finger must be dealt with, but it does not require mobilization of all the individual's defense mechanisms. The inflammatory process is, in actuality, the body's localized response to injury.

The purpose of the inflammatory process is to repel or destroy any invaders and to mend the local damaged area. This process will be activated for such internal stressors as ulceration of the stomach lining or external stressors such as a bee sting. The complex of behaviors comprising this defense mechanism is listed here so that the reader can visualize the changes in the behavioral features and actions that he would identify. The reader must keep in mind that these same behaviors will occur regardless of the stressor. A cut, a burn, or turning an ankle will each activate the same response. The underlying behavioral responses are as follows:

1. Dilation of the blood vessels in the localized area so that there is more blood flowing through that area.
2. Alteration of vascular cell wall membranes so that fluid and white blood cells can shift from the bloodstream into the interstitial spaces.
3. Proliferation of connective tissue in order to wall off the area and prevent the spread of invading organisms.
4. Secretion of chemical substances to neutralize the poisons, kill the bacteria, and expunge or absorb destroyed materials.
5. Granulation or filling in of the area if tissue integrity is disrupted.

The nurse would make the following behavioral observations:

1. The area may be warm to the touch because of the increased blood flow in the area.
2. Skin may be pink or red, reflecting the vasodilation if the injury is near the skin surface.
3. Swelling or edema may be noted as a result of the engorgement of the surrounding tissue.
4. The patient may have pain that occurs when the increased fluid in the area causes pressure against the nerve endings, as well as pain resulting from direct trauma to the nerve endings caused by the injury itself.
5. Because of the pain, the patient may restrict or alter the usual movement of the involved part.
6. Abscess or palpable mass resulting from the accumulation of pus may be observed.

A person may not even be aware of the activation of the underlying inflammatory process unless he has some degree of pain or discomfort. For example, the localized defense process will usually resolve the appendicitis situation several times before its adaptive capacity is exhausted. If and when the localized response to the stressor is unsuccessful, the general systemic activity will be increased and vigorous and extensive behavioral changes will ensue.

The generalized defense responses must be mobilized when more tissue mass becomes involved and cellular breakdown products escape from the local area. In effect, the toxins or cellular breakdown products escape the local area and spread to other parts of the body through the lymphatic system and the bloodstream. Other localized inflammatory processes are initiated in many places throughout the body, with extensive vascular dilation and loss of vascular wall integrity leading to fluid shifting from the bloodstream into the interstitial spaces. If this process, now maladaptive, continues unchecked, it finally leads to total circulatory collapse.

The endocrine system responds before this point, however, by increased secretion of antidiuretic hormones (ADH), mineralocorticoids, and glucocorticoids.* The ADH and the mineralocorticoids reestablish the proper relationship of the vascular blood volume to the increased vascular capacity by effecting renal retention of water and salts. The glucocorticoids act directly on the cell membranes of the vascular system to reduce vascular permeability and maintain vascular tone. Additionally, the automatic regulatory mechanisms of the autonomic nervous system are called into play.

Autonomic nervous system

The autonomic nervous system has two divisions: the parasympathetic and the sympathetic. With exceptions, both of these divisions innervate the same organs. (See Fig. 14.) The divisions are structured in such a way that the parasympathetic division can exert an effect on a single organ without disturbing the other organs it innervates, while the sympathetic division usually stimulates changes simultaneously in all the organs that it innervates. This structuring allows a wide variation in responses to changes in either the internal or external environments.

The ordinary day-to-day maintenance activities usually call for singular and isolated adjustments. These maintenance activities have been referred to as the "vegetative" or "feed-and-breed" activities. The parasympathetic division has the responsibility for these ongoing adjustments, and generally these adjustments are not obvious at the organismic level as long as the range of activity does not exceed the parameters of the steady state.

There are, however, many times during a day when singular and isolated adjustments will not meet the demands of the situation, times when a more all-encompassing activity is required. Any event that requires sudden or extreme alteration in the internal environment will require massive, coordinated responses. A quick dash to the car, a sudden joyous occasion, a passionate kiss, or a sudden change in environmental temperature are examples of events that call for widespread and simultaneous physiologic changes. For instance, a game of tennis will call for massive, simultaneous changes in order to readjust the internal milieu to meet the increased demands at that time. The vigorous sympathetic activity will immediately be reflected by changes in behavior at the observable organismic level. This latter fact

---

*The essential point for students who have not had a physiology course yet is that the endocrine system alters the cellular processes in such a way that the now nonproductive inflammatory process is deactivated.

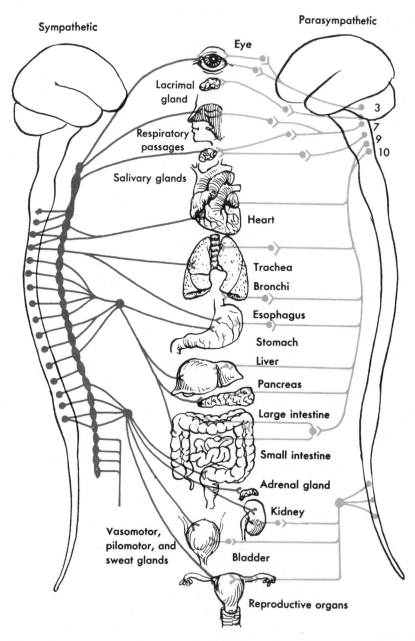

Sympathetic

Parasympathetic

Eye

Lacrimal gland

Respiratory passages

Salivary glands

Heart

Trachea

Bronchi

Esophagus

Stomach

Liver

Pancreas

Large intestine

Small intestine

Adrenal gland

Kidney

Vasomotor, pilomotor, and sweat glands

Bladder

Reproductive organs

3
7
9
10

Fig. 14. Diagram of the autonomic nervous system. The craniosacral (parasympathetic) division is shown in gray. The thoracolumbar (sympathetic) division is shown in red. (From Bergersen, Betty S., and Goth, A.: Pharmacology in nursing, ed. 13, St. Louis, 1976, The C. V. Mosby Co.)

explains why there are groups or clusters of symptoms that the nurse will observe when the protective mechanisms have been activated.

Although we will use the words *emergency* and *crisis,* we quickly reemphasize that the defense responses are activated in many situations that we don't think of in the emergency or crisis category. A *crisis* situation might better be defined as *any unusual, extreme, or threatening situation that calls for immediate resolution of the stressors or a reallocation of energies so that adaptation can occur.* The nurse must also remember that whether the crisis is real or simply perceived as real, the automatic defense mechanisms will be activated because the person's thoughts and feelings can affect the autonomic nervous system activity.

In a crisis situation, the internal physiologic regulatory mechanisms prepare Man for fight or flight, and the body in essence goes into a ready-alert status. The person usually becomes more alert and able to cope with the stressors. The ready-alert behaviors are called nonspecific because they constitute a group of responses that will occur regardless of the stressor. The stressor may be a physical agent such as cold, heat, radiation, infectious agent, mechanical trauma, forced muscular exercise, hemorrhage, pain, fear, or intense emotional involvement. The behaviors themselves are very specific in purpose but are categorized as nonspecific with reference to their cause. The following complex of behaviors are *some* of the underlying changes occurring:

1. Cardiovascular output is increased.
2. The blood flow to the skin, kidney, and other organs not essential for immediate survival is decreased to ensure the ready supply to the more vital areas such as the brain and skeletal and heart muscles.
3. Nonessential functions such as digestion and excretion are slowed down.
4. Salt and water are retained by the kidneys to bolster the blood volume.
5. Muscle tone is increased.
6. Close vision becomes more acute and pupils dilate so that the maximum light can be used in viewing the situation.
7. Respiratory rate and depth are increased to ensure adequate oxygenation of the blood.
8. Metabolism is increased to provide for immediate energy.
9. Since heat is a by-product of metabolism, mechanisms to aid in heat dissipation are often activated.

When the body is presented with an event or condition that calls for vigorous, widespread, and immediate action, the sympathetic division activity is intensified. The nurse might expect to see the following deviation in organismic behavior reflecting the underlying processes:

> **Pupils:** may be dilated.
> **Skin:** may be pale or ashen color, cool to touch, palms of hands "clammy" with perspiration.

Nailbeds: may be pale, lacking usual pinkness.

Mouth: may describe "dry mouth"; lips may be pale in color.

Pulse: may be more rapid than usual; has feeling of full volume to the touch.

Blood pressure: may be elevated.

Stomach: may have lack of appetite.

Intestinal tract: may be unable to defecate; may describe "gas pains" caused by retention of flatus (gas); abdomen may be distended.

Urinary tract: may be unable to void or may indicate urge to urinate but have only small amounts of urine.

Skeletal muscles: activities may be very coordinated and precise or may note rigidity and tremors.

Respiration: depth and rate of respirations may increase; may note use of accessory neck and abdominal muscles in breathing.

Temperature: may be elevated.

Pain: reaction to pain may be reduced for a short time.

Intellectual processes: ability to preceive relevant data and problem solving may be increased.

The words *may be* preface each of the preceding observations to indicate that the nurse might observe some or all of the potential deviations. The individual's organ system idiosyncrasies and the fact that his thoughts and feelings influence his responses lead to a great deal of individual variation.

There are also times when *parts* of the parasympathetic division are inadvertently stimulated in a crisis because of the proximity of the parasympathetic and sympathetic division nerve fibers. Consequently, when stress intensifies, there may be *some* behaviors that are the opposite of those listed under the sympathetic division. Should the parasympathetic division inadvertently stimulate *all* the organs that it innervates at the same time, there would be massive behavioral disorganization. The range of possible deviations observed at the organismic level is much broader than the preceding discussion would indicate. The nurse may expect to see:

Pupils: may be constricted instead of dilated.

Pulse: may be slow and thready instead of rapid and full.

Blood pressure: may drop instead of elevating.

Mouth: may have excessive secretion of saliva instead of dry mouth.

Stomach: nausea and vomiting; feelings of hunger or "hunger pangs" instead of lack of appetite.

Intestinal tract: involuntary defecation or diarrhea.

Urinary tract: involuntary urination.

Intellectual processes: may be unable to focus and think extending to unconsciousness if blood pressure drops sufficiently.

It is not necessary for the nurse to attempt to categorize the origin of the observed behavioral deviations as either parasympathetic, sympathetic, or endocrine responses. It is vital, however, that the nurse be aware of the possible range of deviation indicating that the general nature or rate of activity of the underlying processes has changed. These changes could mean that more energy is being expended to maintain a steady state or that the limits of the steady state have been exceeded.

A NURSING ASSESSMENT OF THE STRESS STATE

We have concluded that when stress intensifies, a person's behavioral stability is likely to become precarious. We have indicated that the stress state intensifies when there is an imbalance between environmental demands (either external or internal) and a person's adaptive capacity. People use a variety of behavioral maneuvers when they are coping with a stressor in an attempt to resolve this imbalance. Reallocation of energy most often is not recognized at a conscious level, so a person is frequently unaware of the behavioral changes instituted to correct or to adjust to the imbalance. The behavioral changes represent a reallocation of his energies. Sometimes they are adaptive, but, unfortunately, at other times they are maladaptive. If the nurse examines a patient's behavior, she may identify some of these changes and therefore be able to estimate the intensity of the stress state as well as the individual's ability to utilize his adaptive capacities.

Six behavioral categories will be presented that represent the behavioral changes commonly occurring when the stress state intensifies. The impetus for such categorization originated with Kurt Lewin's work reported by Leitch and Escalona[9] in 1949 and in the nursing literature by Dorothy E. Johnson[10] in 1961. We will present a delineation and description of six assessment categories that have helped students to make more thorough and definitive observations in an organized manner. The categorization encompasses the wide variety of deviations that may occur when the limits of the steady state are exceeded. Although the same behavior may be indicative of more than one category, we do not believe that this detracts from the usefulness of this tool.

It should be emphasized that the foundation for these assessment categories has been laid by all the content in the preceding chapters. In particular, these categories interrelate the material of Chapter 2 and of the preceding section of this chapter. When observing a person as a unified whole, the nurse will examine both the voluntary regulatory behaviors and the surface deviations reflecting alterations in the automatic activity of the subsystems. The nurse will attempt to determine the regularity and constancy of the patient's usual behavioral patterns and then measure his current conduct against his previous norms. The consistency, coherency, and orderliness of his behaviors give clues as to the effectiveness and efficiency of this functioning, so that the nurse is able to estimate the patient's location on the behavioral stability continuum. Thus, the predictability factors of Man's behavior become a useful tool for the nursing assessment of the stress state.

The six assessment categories are as follows:
1. Accentuated use of one mode or pattern of behavior
2. Alteration in the variety of activities usually undertaken
3. Behavior that is less organized or organized at a lower level of behavioral organization
4. Demonstration of greater sensitivity to the environment
5. Presence of behaviors reflecting alteration in usual physiologic activity
6. Distortion of "reality"

Before discussing each of the assessment categories in more detail, it is essential that four points be established. First, the nurse must remember that regardless of whether the change is adaptive or maladaptive, it may be a clue that the stress state has intensified.

Second, often the nurse will not know the person before he becomes a patient. Although the nurse has a background reservoir of generalizations about patterns of daily living activities and knowledge of deviations reflecting changes in the underlying physiologic processes, these generalizations are only a starting point. Unfortunately, there are times when the nurse has little or no time to establish an individual's previous baseline before intervention is required. For instance, the nurse and the doctor must act quickly when a critically injured patient is admitted via the emergency room, and even the characteristics of his structural variable profile may not be completely identified. A situation also becomes more complicated when a language barrier exists. There will be times when the nurse must necessarily depend upon the generalizations or norms for a similar person in a comparable situation until he or she is able to secure more adequate individual patient data.

Third, there are some behaviors so commonly associated with intensification of stress that there is a danger that a nurse may accept them at face value without questioning the validity of her conclusions. Purposeless behaviors such as finger tapping, hair twirling, pacing the floor, and nail biting are often positively correlated with an intensification of the stress state. Many times, however, these behaviors have become so habitualized over a period of years that they are no longer significant indices of the stress state for an individual. Only by observing the patient for a time or by talking with the patient, his physician, his family, or his friends will the nurse be able to judge adequately whether this behavior is a valid index of the severity of the stress state.

Fourth, the nurse must keep in mind that the absence of clues of an intensified stress state at the organismic level may not mean that the activity is within the limits of the steady state. In the resistance phase (see Fig. 13, p. 75) it was indicated that the level of resistance is considerably higher than usual. In this phase there may be no overt behavioral cues because the patient is coping or adjusting to the stress. However, he is utilizing a great deal more energy in his adaptation at this time than in the prestressor period. He will continue to do so until the environmental situation is rectified, or he will eventually enter the exhaustion phase as his adaptive capacity becomes depleted.

A young woman with two children who displays little grief after the death of her husband may be an example of the preceding situation. The relative and community groups may praise her ''courage and internal fortitude'' when she quickly readjusts her life and carries on as if the death were not a crisis. These people may overlook the precariousness of the widow's behavioral stability because they see her adjusting well in the visible aspects of her life situation. They don't realize that if she has simply repressed her feelings, the widow would not be allocating her energies appropriately and working toward resolution of the stressor. The grief and mourning process, which entails an awareness of her feelings and appropriate release of them, is critical for reestablishment of her steady state. Denial or repression of the natural feelings of guilt and loss utilize energy, and she may be in a state of precarious behavioral stability even though there may be little evidence of the intensified stress state.

A more ordinary example occurred recently in a clinical laboratory setting. A student who was doing ''A'' work said to her instructor: ''You know, I'm so nervous and scared when I'm starting a new procedure, but all the other students think that I am very calm and collected. They keep asking me for help, and they do not realize how hard it is for me.'' Frequently, in everyday life, outward calmness is mistaken for an indication of the steady state.

There are times when, by virtue of knowing the stressor or potential stressor, the nurse knows that not having an increase in stress would be extremely unusual. If a patient entered the hospital for surgery, the nurse would be more concerned about him if he did not have any manifestation of an intensified stress state than if he did.* If the nurse cannot identify some plausible reason that explains the lack of cues, the patient would be dealt with as though he were manifesting behavioral clues of stress, because the patient cannot maintain the resistance phase indefinitely. The absence of behavioral cues, in the presence of an obvious stressor, does not mean that there is not an intensification of the stress state. It may mean that the person is utilizing a great deal of energy in such an adaptation. If the nurse has reason to suspect that the patient is adapting to the stressor without resolution of the stressor itself, intervention must be initiated to assist the patient to put the stressor into its proper perspective.

Having made four preliminary precautionary comments, we will now turn to a discussion of the six assessment categories that may indicate an intensification of stress.

---

*Janis has done some interesting research on pre- and postoperative surgical patients that illustrates this point.[11]

Accentuated use of one mode or pattern of behavior

Intensification of stress may be reflected by a more pronounced utilization of a behavior or group of behaviors that constitutes one or more of the individual's usual behavioral patterns. This pronounced usage may be a cue that the person is expending more energy than usual in attempting to maintain or regain his steady state. Therefore, the nurse will observe for some particular behavior or group of behaviors that has become more prominent or conspicuous in its usage. A person may nibble on foods at intervals throughout the day, but when the stress state has intensified, he may be observed eating almost constantly. A jolly person who ordinarily laughs a lot may be noticed laughing when it is not appropriate. A man who laughs when he is told that his surgical incision must be reopened and drained may be camouflaging his real feelings, both from himself and from others. Some people attempt to maintain a semblance of order by adhering to their usual patterns, even though they may no longer serve a useful purpose. This person may be observed adhering more rigidly to his usual schedule or method of doing things. Thus, observation of accentuated use of one behavior or pattern of behavior may indicate that the individual's stress state has exceeded the limits of the steady state.

Alteration in the variety of activities usually undertaken

One method by which some people reallocate their energies is to decrease the variety of activities usually undertaken, which releases some of their energies for other uses. An individual who habitually snacks regularly throughout the day may lose all interest in snacking, or even food in general, when his stress state is intensified. A student who is concerned about an examination may not do dishes, or make the bed, or keep her customary evening date in order to concentrate on her studies before an examination. To put these observations into context, however, the student's usual patterns must be considered; perhaps she rarely does dishes until the clean supply is exhausted, and the bed may be made only when the sheets are changed once a week.

In the hospital, the nurse might become concerned about a woman who has been carefully grooming herself and suddenly stops, since this may be a cue that there is a new stressor, either real or perceived, with which she is having difficulty. A person may usually watch television or read whenever he has time to do so, yet when hospitalized may show no interest in either for several days after admittance. Many times, the first clue that the nurse will identify that indicates that the patient is finally beginning to feel better is a request for a comb, lipstick, or razor or for the television to be turned on. These people are resuming activities that had been deleted because of the severity of the stress state.

Other people reallocate their energies by undertaking more than their usual variety of activities. It must be recognized that when the stress state intensifies, *some* people respond by monitoring their energy allocation more carefully than under ordinary circumstances. Therefore, these people will remain well organized, and the increase in variation of their activities will enable them to cope with the stressor. A mother of a child who was terminally ill, in addition to her usual home activities, care of her husband, and frequent visiting in the hospital, managed to work with the cancer society's fund-raising activities.

Thus, a person may attempt to cope with stressors by deviating from his customary routines; he may either decrease or increase the variety of activities he undertakes.

Behavior that is less organized or organized at a lower level of behavioral organization

All people organize themselves in their environment at a particular organizational level depending upon their age and stage of development. The extent of organization at that level will vary from individual to individual. When the stress state intensifies, the nurse may be able to identify clues that the patient has deviated either from his usual degree of organization, or in the level at which his behavior is organized.

The disorganization factor reflects a difficulty in apportioning of energy. It is usually identified by noting behaviors that lack appropriate priority or inappropriate attention to detail or those activities that utilize energy with no other purpose.* There are two examples that illustrate the inappropriate priority or attention to detail. A student who rushes off to take an examination may well forget to take either her purse or a pen. Frequently, a student making her first home visit in community nursing leaves the office without the nursing bag that has just been prepared. There are times when a person does not know how or is unable to utilize his energies in a constructive fashion. The nurse in this case may observe very purposeless activities, such as blinking eyes, miscellaneous hand or leg movements, lip chewing, pacing the floor, or rambling pointless verbalization. The nurse must attempt to make a distinction between those purposeless or rhythmic movements that occur as a manifestation of the stress state and those that have become habitualized. As indicated earlier, a habit such as nail biting may be a behavior that occurs regularly regardless of the individual's stress state.

The level of behavioral organization is the second factor that the nurse must con-

---

*Purposeless activities were considered as a separate category entitled "Breakdown in Economy of Action" by K. Lewin and discussed by D. Johnson.[10] The authors found that students became confused because they often could not distinguish between a behavior that was "disorganized" and one that was "purposeless." The students would, however, correlate the assessment categories and their clinical observations very meaningfully when purposeless activity was considered under the organizational category presented here.

sider. Sometimes people will revert to behaviors that were associated with an earlier stage of their development but that are out of character at the current stage. A hospitalized child who sucks his thumb—something that he may not have been doing for 3 or 4 years—is an example of a behavior indicative of a lower level of behavioral organization. Another classic example is frequently observed following the arrival of a new sibling into the home. At this time, the older child who was toilet trained may revert to wetting his pants or demanding to be fed once again by the bottle. The nurse may observe an adult who is exhibiting very dependent behavior; he may be unable to make a decision about even the simplest activities without consultation with the staff. This person may be employed as a top echelon business executive responsible for major decisions yet, in this instance, be incapacitated as a result of the degree of stress. A 50-year-old woman may be exhibiting very coquettish behavior with any man encountered; however, the nurse would not judge this one piece of information by itself—it would have to be supported by many other cues before a judgment would be made about this woman's stress status.

Demonstration of greater sensitivity to the environment

Sometimes, when the stress state is intensified, a person just does not have enough energy left to cope with even the usual environmental input. Environmental changes or events that normally have had little significance for him may develop into critical issues, and frequently his responses are out of proportion to the stressor itself. The person's tolerance level, in general, is decreased to the point where things that usually don't bother him become very annoying. Light, which would usually not be bothersome to an individual, may be very irritating. Noises of which the nurses may not even be aware can be annoying to a patient who, under other circumstances, would not notice them either. Changes in room temperature or wind flow are frequently stressors to a person who is ill, yet at other times he would not be aware or speak of them. The traffic flow and seating arrangements in an outpatient clinic can be extremely aggravating to a person who has returned for his first postdischarge examination. The nurse must recognize the irritation over seemingly minor things may be an indication of an intensified stress state.

Presence of behaviors reflecting alteration in usual physiologic activity

The nurse must think through the behaviors that are automatically instituted to prepare Man for "fight or flight," since they also represent an alteration in energy allocation. The nurse would carefully examine the shell that houses Man for changes in behavioral features that reflect the status of the underlying behaviors. She would observe such behavioral features as skin and nailbed coloration, pupillary changes, pulse rate, depth and rate of respiration, both quality and quantity of verbalization, and voice pitch and volume. (See list on pp. 81-82.) The nurse would, of course, supplement her observational senses by use of such instruments as thermometers or blood pressure apparatus to extend observation below the surface.

The nurse must recognize that when the stress state exceeds the limits of the steady state, Man's subsystems become more sensitive to external environmental changes. The thoughts and feelings of a person will have greater potential to influence the coordination and integration of the subsystem activity. We doubt that any reader has not experienced a sudden urge to void before a test or an exciting date, even though he may have voided twice within the past hour. Fear and excitement may also result in diarrhea or nausea. We can even say that the bowel, bladder, and stomach organs tend to lose their autonomy in the presence of an intensified stress state.

Distortion of "reality"

There are many times when an individual's energy allocation affects his intellectual processes and his problem-solving ability may be decreased. When the stress state intensifies, a person's thought processes may become so altered that he is not logically thinking something through to its obvious conclusion. He may not be incorporating all the facts into his thought processes or, indeed, he may actually not "hear" what has been said. He may have difficulty determining what are the relevant data in his situation or in using appropriately the data that he already has at his disposal. His system of priorities may become distorted because he cannot accurately attach meaning to the input stimuli.

An individual may misinterpret or misunderstand what to others is a perfectly normal event. A nurse caring for a group of patients was observed by one of those patients with a syringe in her hand. He immediately became very upset, thinking that he was going to receive an injection. Later on, when he saw the nurse put a "nothing by mouth" sign above his bed, he immediately concluded that he was going to have surgery. Another patient who had had a vein stripping was told that she must keep her leg elevated and she indicated to the roommate that this meant that the surgery had failed.

During the course of any day, a student will encounter many examples of distortion of reality that may reflect an intensification of the stress state. Distortion may occur because a person does not realistically perceive either the stressor or his own adaptive capacities. Consequently, distortion of reality can be a common and natural phenomenon when stress is intensified and should not automatically be labeled pathologic.

The preceding six assessment categories provide a logical and comprehensive method for data gathering. Once all of the behavioral data have been gathered, they must be evaluated in their totality. There may be a large number of minor changes noted in each category, or there may be a large number of major importance. There may be only a few changes in one category, but they may be of major significance. The nurse must recognize that there is a wide range in normalcy. Obviously, however, if a person's behavior continuously or consistently reflects one or all of these categories, it may be indicative of psychophysiopathology. The implications that will be drawn will depend upon the factors involved in the particular situation and are beyond the scope of this book. We have provided a means for assessment that we believe is a helpful approach to the assessment of the stress state.

SUMMARY

Stress is essential for life, and it is always present to some degree because adjustments are continually being made to internal and external environmental changes. When the activities involved in these adjustments (either voluntary or automatic) exceed the limits of the steady state, the patient's behavioral stability may become precarious. When this occurs, there usually will be observable manifestations in a person's behavior features and actions.

The results of a person's adjustments may be either adaptive or maladaptive for him as a unified whole. Since moderate intensification of the stress state serves a constructive purpose for an individual's growth and learning, maladaptation results only when the individual's adaptive capacities are reduced to the point where he no longer has the resources to regain the steady state without assistance.

Intensification of the stress state has three phases. In the alarm phase, the person perceives a stressor and initiates action to mobilize his defenses. In the resistance phase, hopefully, adaptation occurs and the process is reversed. If it is not, the exhaustion phase is entered when the individual's adaptive capacities have become overtaxed. Since energy resources are limited, external aids must sometimes be provided. The nurse must be able to analyze both the demands made of the patient by his daily activities and his adaptive capacities as an integrated behavioral unit.

The stressor itself must be evaluated. This is done by considering the nature and the number of stressors involved, the duration or anticipated duration of exposure, and the person's past experiences with a comparable stressor. The nurse must be concerned with potential stressors, as well as those currently present, because their effects may be avoided or ameliorated by nursing intervention. It must be remembered that when the stress state intensifies, the state itself can become a stressor to the person.

The nurse knows that when the subsystem's defense mechanisms are activated, there will be groups of responses that will occur simultaneously when the individual perceives a novel or injurious stressor. These physiologic behaviors are reflected by changes in the organismic behavioral features and actions of the patient. Therefore, the nurse will note any deviations in the characteristic behavioral features of the shell that houses Man. The nurse also knows that the nature and degree of alteration in the usual patterned activities of daily living may provide cues of the stress status. Most important of all, the nurse knows that the presence of clues may or may not give valid estimation of the stress state's intensity and, conversely, knows that neither can the absence of behavioral clues be equated with the steady state.

By using the six assessment categories presented in this chapter, some estimation can be made regarding the severity of the stress state and the patient's ability to adjust in his daily living. The nurse will base a determination of the stress state on careful observation of the deviations in the patient's usual patterns of daily living and the deviations that imply intensification of the activity at the subsystem level. Only after carefully observing the patient's behavioral features and actions and comparing them with his previous baseline will the nurse be in a position to make the soundest possible judgments regarding the patient's adaptive status. There are times, however, when the nurse will be forced to rely on generalizations for a person with a similar structural variable profile in a comparable situation until adequate information can be gathered about the specific patient.

We have introduced the stress concept and suggested a framework for making definitive and comprehensive observation of the stress state. Subsequent courses and texts will amplify this concept both in theory and in practical application in all clinical areas.

REFERENCES

1. Selye, Hans: The stress of life, New York, 1956, McGraw-Hill Book Co.
2. Lazarus, R. S.: Psychological stress and the coping process, New York, 1956, McGraw-Hill Book Co., chap. 10.
3. Weitz, J.: Stress, research paper (IDA/HQ 66-4762), Institute for Defense Analysis, April, 1966, p. 521.
4. Appley, M. H., and Trumbull, R.: Psychological stress, New York, 1967, Appleton-Century-Crofts.
5. Mountcastle, V. B., editor: Medical physiology, ed. 12, St. Louis, 1968, The C. V. Mosby Co., pp. 176, 923, 985-988, 1091, 1147.
6. McGrath, J. E., editor: Social and psychological factors in stress, New York, 1970, Holt, Rinehart, & Winston, Inc., chaps. 1, 2, 9.
7. Kahn, R. L., and others: Organizational stress: studies in role conflict and ambiguity, New York, 1964, John Wiley & Sons, Inc., chap. 6.
8. Selye, Hans: The stress syndrome, American Journal of Nursing **65:**98, 1965.
9. Leitch, M., and Escalona, S.: Reactions of infants to stress, Psychoanalytic Study of the Child **3-4:**121-140, 1949.
10. Johnson, Dorothy E.: The significance of nursing care, American Journal of Nursing **61:**63-66, 1961.
11. Janis, I. L.: Stress: psychoanalytic and behavioral studies of surgical patients, New York, 1958, John Wiley & Sons, Inc., chap. 22.

ADDITIONAL READINGS

Bajusz, Ecors, editor: Physiology and pathology of adaptive mechanisms: neural-neuroendocrine-humoral, New York, 1969, Pergamon Press, Inc.

Cannon, Walter B.: The wisdom of the body, New York, 1932, W. W. Norton & Co.

Grossman, S. B.: A textbook of physiological psychology, New York, 1967, John Wiley & Sons, Inc.

Guyton, Arthur C.: Function of the human body, Philadelphia, 1969, W. B. Saunders Co.

Langeley, L. L.: Homeostasis, New York, 1965, Van Nostrand Reinhold Co.

Menninger, Karl, Mayman, Martin, and Pruyser, Paul: The vital balance, New York, 1963, The Viking Press, Inc.

Woodburne, L. S.: The neural basis of behavior, Columbus, Ohio, 1967, Charles E. Merrill Publishing Co.

Chapter 7

A PERSPECTIVE FOR PREDICTION OF CONSEQUENCES

This chapter will be devoted to an examination of the idea that *an act has more than one consequence,* and this notion will be treated as a rudimentary key concept for both the study and the practice of nursing. Exploration of this concept should enable the student to define clearly the anticipated outcome for nursing activities and to evaluate the outcomes actually achieved. Since Man has a limited amount of energy available for the adaptive process, it is essential that the nurse make every activity or nurse-patient interaction as productive as possible, so that energy is allocated in such a way that the steady state can be maintained or regained and cure can take place. An activity or task has no one single outcome. Therefore, nurses can enhance their interactions if they consciously take advantage of all the possible ends that can be achieved with a single action.

The average person is accustomed to thinking about only one reason why he undertakes an activity or course of action. That is to say, he is usually consciously aware of only the main outcome or end he hopes to achieve. Although he may be vaguely aware that other consequences transpire as a result of his undertaking, he most often accepts them matter of factly and without conscious consideration. Most people, if questioned and given time to think about it, could identify a number of consequences that result from any one of their activities. Ordinarily, however, they take them for granted and only stop to review them when a negative consequence becomes apparent or when they are unable to achieve the desired end or goal. Moreover, when people begin to take the outcomes for granted, they also begin to view the activity as an end in and of itself, rather than as a means to an end or variety of outcomes.

This orientation or general life-style is often carried over into the practice of nursing without the person's realization. Frequently, the person who is embarking upon a career in nursing considers giving injections, enemas, taking vital signs, and other procedures as defining the full scope of "nursing." He or she wants to learn how and when to do the various procedures and views these activities as ends in

93

and of themselves. Some of the actions or activities carried out for patients might be considered unnecessary, or even menial, unless the nurse understands the concept that an act has more than one consequence and learns to consider and predict what these consequences will be.

The all-too-common practice of looking at patient care as a series of procedures to be completed places the emphasis on the task itself rather than on the patient and his adaptive processes. This practice has prompted many authors to write about the necessity for a patient-centered focus for nursing care. Incorporation of the concept that an act has more than one consequence into daily practice will keep the nurse from falling into the trap of routinized care with the activity itself as the end, rather than the means to a variety of ends. The emphasis on outcomes to be achieved will ensure a patient-centered focus for nursing activities and will enable the nurse to maximize the effectiveness of procedures and routines carried out with and on behalf of the patient.

The nurse must be *consciously* aware of as many potential consequences as it is possible to identify. Before undertaking any activity with the patient, there are three questions the nurse must answer that will lead to *overt* awareness of the full scope of the consequences to be anticipated. The three questions are:

1. For whom does the activity have consequences?
2. What are the consequences that can be anticipated?
3. What is the value of the consequences for those involved?

Each of these questions will be discussed in detail in order that the full impact of each question will be clearly understood.

FOR WHOM DOES THE ACTIVITY HAVE CONSEQUENCES?

Consequences for the patient, who is the recipient of nursing care, would most certainly be considered. There appears to be a certain reluctance to acknowledge that the "doer," in this case the nurse, is affected by the same activity. Nursing students who enter the profession with the popular lay image of the nurse as a self-giving, self-denying, dedicated individual often find if difficult to consider the consequences for themselves that result from their patient care activities. There are consequences for the nurse, however, and these consequences often directly affect future intervention with patients. If a patient is friendly and tries hard to do his deep-breathing exercises as taught by the nurse, the nurse has a feeling of reward for the effort expended. Because of these positive feelings, the nurse may stop in the patient's room to check on his progress very frequently. On the other hand, a nurse who feels helpless in the face of a terminal illness will frequently avoid the patient who is dying, thus reinforcing that patient's feelings of isolation. A nurse who has to turn a patient in pain may avoid doing a complete job because of feelings of sympathy and guilt aroused because she is causing the patient to experience a more intense pain. The nurse who has carefully identified all the ends to be achieved by nursing intervention will be in a much better position to deal with her own feelings. Thus, consequences for the nurse as well as for the patient must be identified in order to ensure that the nurse will be able to make the most effective use of self in nurse-patient interactions.

Additionally, an activity usually has consequences for other people in the patient's universe. This fact is not commonly or often consciously considered. These other persons may be other staff members, family members, co-workers, or friends. The patient's behavior affects the responses of any "significant others" and, in turn, their response will affect him.

If the nurse gives a pain injection just before visiting hours, the patient is more comfortable for a period of time. When the visitors arrive, they consequently will be relieved since they usually conclude that the patient is really making excellent progress. Sometimes negative results will occur if the visitors make more demands of him because of their postinjection observations. They may expect consultation on work or family home problems, lengthen their visit, or nonverbally encourage the patient's involvement in social interaction with them, which utilizes more energy than he can afford to use. Their expectations for his behavior or their actions can leave the patient totally exhausted following the visit. The nurse who considers consequences of the injection for "others" would most likely either anticipate the need for intervention by talking with the visitors before they enter the room, or later during the visit by assessing the patient's status and speaking with the visitors if the situation then requires it.

The same kind of situation arises with the doctors and visitors following the "AM bath." Clean ironed sheets, combed hair, and lipstick applied by the nurse may totally distort the true picture. The patient may have had a miserable 24-hour period, with the overt misery being erased by the clean sheets, shave, or application of cosmetics. The doctor might decide to change his orders based on that appraisal following the AM care visit, and it is possible that the pain medication dosage might be altered prematurely.

Too often nurses don't capitalize on the fact that the "significant others" do not need to be present to be affected by a nurse-patient activity. The following example is used to illustrate a situation where the outcomes for an absent family member, anticipated by the nurse, were actually achieved even though the nurse did not meet the patient's husband because he worked during her shift. A nurse was working with a woman who had a long leg cast applied because of a fractured tibia. The nurse explained muscle setting exercises and the reasons why Mrs. S. needed to put all the uninvolved joints and muscles through complete range of motion while in the hospital. She then extended the discussion to the need for a regular and complete range of motion exercise regimen as part of everyone's daily activities. As they talked, Mrs. S. suddenly said: "My husband and I have been arguing because he wants to play handball twice a week. Perhaps I shouldn't be upset since he sits at a desk all day and our social activities are primarily sitting activities. Although he is having fun without me, his muscles really need the exercise." Several weeks later the nurse passed Mrs. S. in the out-patient clinic. Mrs. S. commented with a smile that she had encouraged her husband to play handball and that when the doctor said it was all right, they planned to take tennis lessons. Since nurses are concerned with assisting all people to attain the highest possible level of wellness, they will utilize every appropriate interaction to disseminate information that will assist people to maximize their potential capabilities. When talking with patients, the nurse can frequently broaden the scope of their discussion to include the family members or involved friends, as occurred in the case of the nurse and Mrs. S. These others need not be physically present to benefit from a nurse-patient interaction.

In summary, those for whom the activity has consequences would include the patient, the nurse herself, other nursing staff or other health team members, and any involved "significant others." The nurse will not limit the identification of consequences to those people who are physically present at the time.

WHAT ARE THE CONSEQUENCES THAT CAN BE ANTICIPATED?

Because Man is an integrated behavioral unit, there are always several consequences associated with any activity. Whenever possible, the nurse will assist the patient with his activities of daily living in such a way as to support both the underlying physiologic behavioral processes and the family or peer group of which the patient is a part. The nurse might encourage a patient to walk to the bathroom, knowing that this act on his part will help him to maintain the muscular tone of his legs and allow blood flow to the pressure areas of his back. The nurse also knows that the experience or knowledge that he has been on his feet reassures both the patient and his family that he is indeed "making progress."

If we are asked to anticipate possible outcomes of a business executive playing volleyball twice a week, the following are some of the associated outcomes, representing various behavioral levels, that might be listed. He will:

1. Enjoy a competitive game
2. Develop blisters on his heels
3. Improve the tone of muscles not ordinarily used
4. Feel more relaxed since he has a legitimate outlet for the aggressive feeling he has been "sitting on"
5. Enlarge his circle of acquaintances and friends
6. Control his weight gain since he is expending more calories than he is ingesting

The reader could also list several possible outcomes that might be anticipated for the wife of the businessman or his co-workers if the "others" for whom this activity had consequences were to be listed.

The nurse is in a position to predict outcomes with greater accuracy if she has knowledge of the cluster of possible outcomes usually associated with a given activity when considering people in general. It is possible to predict a cluster of consequences occurring simultaneously for any activity whether it is giving a backrub, feeding a patient, or having the patient give his own bedbath. Clusters of consequences for nursing procedures or activities that the nurse can anticipate for the majority of people will evolve as more content is presented in the various nursing courses. These "norms" for the cluster of anticipated consequences of a specific activity provide a baseline for planning nursing care for a particular patient. When the nurse meets the patient for the first time it is essential to think through the generalizations that can be made about consequences for a specific activity. The nurse then applies the facts learned about the patient and individualizes the cluster of consequences to be achieved in his care. Some of the usual consequences will need to be maximized and others minimized depending upon the condition and circumstances of the patient.

Even the most proficient nurse will rarely be able to anticipate consequences for a specific patient with total accuracy. The patient's previous experiences and background and the idiosyncrasies of his organ-system operation are often an unknown quantity affecting his responses. Additionally, the multitude of external environmental influences that may act as intervening variables are often difficult to identify, much less control. Application of the generalizations that can be made about consequences for an activity in context with as much knowledge as possible about the patient does markedly increase the probability of the nurse's predictions being correct.

WHAT IS THE VALUE OF THE CONSEQUENCES FOR THOSE INVOLVED?

Once clusters of anticipated outcomes have been identified, the nurse must then decide whether the consequences are adaptive or maladaptive for the specific patient in the stipulated situation. It must be remembered that such judgments are based on knowledge of Man as an organismic unit in context with the information she has acquired about the various behavioral levels *in terms of their contribution to the patient as an ongoing behavioral unit*. The nurse will, of course, collaborate with other health team members when there is a question about consequences within their area of specialization.

A patient who has had surgery and tends to lie in one position may experience less pain than if he moves about in the bed. He is considering only one of the cluster of consequences that is occurring simultaneously as a result of limiting his movement, however. In addition to minimizing the amount of discomfort experienced, limitation of movement may also have the following negative consequences*:

1. Fluid pools in one part of the lungs, which interferes with the oxygen–carbon dioxide exchange
2. Blood supply to the tissues over bony prominences decreases, which leads to tissue death and development of bedsores (decubiti)
3. Muscle tone generally decreases, which leads to weakness and fatigue when attempting to get up or to muscle atrophy seen when "foot-drop" develops
4. Gas (flatus) tends to accumulate in the bowel, which leads to distention and general abdominal discomfort
5. The patient begins to think that it isn't possible for him to move since he does not accurately assess his actual capacity for movement

If there is a medical reason that the patient should not be turned, the physician will so indicate in his written orders on the patient's chart. If there is no such restriction, the nurse will consider all the consequences resulting from limitation of movement and will determine that the negative consequences far outweigh the positive consequence of pain reduction for the patient's total welfare. Therefore, the nurse would be sure that the patient is turned from side to side at regular intervals, recognizing that there are ways of turning patients that will minimize the pain even though it cannot be eliminated entirely.

The simple act of answering a patient's call bell promptly might have the following three positive outcomes: (1) his request for the bedpan will be granted; he urinates and feels more comfortable; (2) he develops trust in the staff since they responded when he needed assistance; and (3) he feels significant as a person rather than an object in a "foreign" environment. If the call bell were not answered immediately, the following negative results might be anticipated. He will: (1) wet his bed or retain the urine, which will lead to decrease in bladder wall muscle tone and potential future difficulty urinating; (2) develop distrust in the staff; and (3) have reinforced his feelings of worthlessness and insignificance in a "foreign" environment.

Let us consider three outcomes that actually occurred when Mr. G. was given an injection for pain: (1) there was a decrease in the amount of discomfort he was experiencing; (2) a rash developed as a manifestation of an allergic reaction to the medication; and (3) his confidence in the doctor was shaken. The nurse is aware that an unusual or negative reaction to a medication is one outcome that is expected for a small percentage of the population and is alert and ready to intervene should an undesirable outcome occur. The nurse is also aware that simultaneously with

---

*These points are included only to illustrate the consequences that can occur in such a situation. Other texts will include study of such complications in depth.

the untoward reaction, the patient may well question the competence of the staff. Anticipating the latter negative consequence, the nurse intervened by pointing out the beneficial actions of the medication and the fact that there was no way of predicting which few persons might have a slightly unfavorable reaction that could be quickly controlled. She indicated that the doctor would want to answer any question or hear any concerns that Mr. G. might have. Later in the day Mr. G. commented to the nurse that he was glad that she had told him about the medication because he had thought that his doctor had just "overlooked something" he should have known about him and the medication, or that the nurse had given him the wrong dose. The nurse's intervention assisted the patient to cope with the minor crisis that had arisen; thus, he utilized less energy in wordless worry and maintained a more optimal tension level.

The nurse must be concerned with the effect of all the consequences for the patient at a specific time. Therefore, she attempts to delete or minimize as many potentially negative consequences as it is possible to control and to capitalize on the potentially positive outcomes *so that the overall complex of consequences has a more positive than negative effect for the patient as an ongoing unit.*

The nurse who is about to give a 2-year-old child a booster DPT (diphtheria, pertussis, tetanus) injection in a child health clinic might anticipate the following outcomes:

1. The body's defenses would be stimulated to develop antibodies to protect the child should he be exposed to diphtheria, whooping cough, or tetanus during the ensuing years.
2. A general reaction might be manifested by elevation of temperature and irritability during the following 3-day period.
3. The child might develop a fear of persons wearing white uniforms, since he associates them with painful and frightening experiences.
4. The child may kick or hit the nurse.

The nurse who anticipates these preceding outcomes establishes a course of action to minimize the negative consequences to the greatest degree possible, so that the overall effect is more positive than negative. The nurse might take the following actions to modify the last two items in the preceding list:

1. Prepare the injection before the child enters the room.
2. Keep the syringe and other equipment out of sight until time to give the injection.
3. Depending upon his age, prepare the child for the slight discomfort by associating the feeling he might anticipate with something with which he is familiar—a mosquito bite, for instance.
4. Position the child so that he cannot harm himself or the nurse when the injection is given.

5. Wear street clothes or various colored uniforms to make the environment less foreign and to avoid the association of a frightening experience with white clothing.
6. Give a small treat to the child as he leaves. A small toy or funny-face mask can do much to end the visit on a pleasant note and to associate some positive feelings with the clinic visit.

UNEXPECTED OUTCOMES

There will be times when an unexpected outcome will become apparent, and the nurse should then attempt to determine its probable cause. If it is a positive outcome, the nurse would like to be able to duplicate the result. If it is negative, the nurse will attempt to control or help the individual to control the events so that the same outcome does not reoccur. The nurse practitioner, by this process, removes her intervention from the realm of intuitive functioning. An astute nurse often can analyze the events preceding the unexpected or puzzling behaviors and identify a probable cause. Of course, an attempt must be made to validate any conclusions with more observational data or discussion with the patient and staff or a review of the literature. Obviously, if the nurse deems that a patient's unexpected behavioral response is inhibiting his progress, it is critical to determine at once what might have prompted his unanticipated or puzzling behavior. Perhaps the nurse will discover that the patient's response is an unanticipated outcome of the nursing intervention itself or resulted from another environmental influence that may be modified. If the causative factor can be pinpointed, the nurse can hopefully supplement the patient's understanding of ''why'' a specific action was taken and may alter the intervention to circumvent the unexpected negative outcome in the future. If the cause is outside the nurse's sphere of control, she will communicate the findings to the appropriate person or persons.

An unexpected outcome once occurred as the result of a head nurse telling a patient who had ''bedrest orders'' that he was not moving enough. The afternoon nurse found the patient sitting on the side of his bed and later that night discovered him in the bathroom. When she attempted to find out why the patient had suddenly started getting out of bed, he stated: ''The 'Boss' nurse told me I was not moving enough.'' This certainly was not an expected or constructive outcome of the head nurse's intervention. The next morning the head nurse spoke with the patient and reinforced the evening nurse's interpretation of her comment regarding his movement. When the patient understood that ''moving enough'' referred only to his position change in bed, he did alternate his position more frequently but made no further attempt to get out of bed. Had the evening nurse simply assumed that the patient was tired of staying in bed and ordered him to remain in bed, he probably would have become angry, had less respect for her, and continued to get up when she was not looking.

ASSESSMENT AND EVALUATION OF CONSEQUENCES

Frequent evaluation must be made because of the rapidly changing nature of the patient's situation. The initial conclusions reached provide the basis for anticipating outcomes and projecting a course of action. It is essential that the outcomes actually achieved be evaluated at intervals and necessary adjustments made. The frequency of reevaluation depends entirely upon the presenting situation. A patient who is having an insulin reaction will need more frequent reevaluation than a stroke patient on a long-term rehabilitation unit. Clinical judgment will be developed by the nurse so that the timing of the evaluation or reassessment is most effective.

Many workers carry out tasks or activities with and on behalf of the patient. In the "reality world" of health care delivery, with all of its conflicting pressures, the nurse will often delegate patient care to ancillary personnel. In the process of identifying consequences to be achieved as a result of nursing service, it must be decided whether only professional personnel should give the care or whether an ancillary worker can be assigned the task with special instructions from the nurse. The ability to assess and specify the individualized goals to be accomplished by the actions and procedures enables the nurse to set the time and the work priorities in the care of various patients.

SUMMARY

We have made the following points about "consequences" in our discussion:
1. There are several outcomes associated with a given activity.
2. The consequences may be of either a positive or a negative value.
3. There may be unexpected outcomes as well as anticipated consequences.
4. The nurse attempts to control the situation so that the overall complex of outcomes for any given activity has a more positive than negative effect for the person as an ongoing functioning unit.
5. Consequences must be reevaluated at frequent intervals depending upon the rapidity of situational change with the achieved outcomes measured against the anticipated outcomes.

The nurses who incorporate the concept that an act has more than one consequence into daily practice will continuously be answering the following three questions:
1. For whom does this activity have consequences?
2. What are the consequences that can be anticipated?
3. What is the value of the consequences for those involved?

The answers to these questions will constantly reinforce just how productive a simple activity can be made by capitalizing on the potential consequences on a conscious level. The nurses who do so will not consider emptying a bedpan, responding to a call bell, or giving a bed bath as menial labor but as their means to achieve a variety of patient-centered goals. They will predict and evaluate a variety of outcomes they hope to achieve or avoid through their activity.

Nurse practitioners can become so proficient in this process that they automatically individualize the range of possible outcomes for a particular patient in a specific situation. Beginning practitioners, however, must make a conscious effort to incorporate this particular step into their thinking in order to ensure the development of awareness and accuracy in their predictions and evaluation of the outcomes as they work with patients.

ADDITIONAL READINGS

Abdellah, Faye G.: Methods of identifying covert aspects of nursing problems, Nursing Research **6**(1):4-27, 1957.

Davis, Ellen: Give a bath? American Journal of Nursing **70**:2366-2367, 1970.

Wiedenback, Ernestine: Nurse's wisdom in nursing theory, American Journal of Nursing **70**:1057-1062, 1970.

Zimmerman, Donna S., and Gohrke, Carol: The goal-directed nursing approach; it does work, American Journal of Nursing **70**:306-310, 1970.

Chapter 8

POSITION AND ROLE
enactment and assessment

Often a person seeking health care is moving into an unfamiliar position; when a person is ill and becomes a patient he has less energy to cope with unfamiliar stressors. The student is also in the process of acquiring a new position, that of a nurse. Both individuals are often uncertain of the behaviors that are appropriate to their newly assumed positions, and this can intensify their stress states. Although they usually have some general ideas or expectations of the role that they must play, these expectations may be neither correct nor complete. Crises can occur because of uncertainties or misconceptions when assuming a new, different, or unfamiliar position.

This chapter introduces two sociologic concepts: position and role. These interrelated concepts are tools the student can use to determine the behaviors meaningful to and appropriately a part of the nurse role as well as those behaviors appropriate to the role of the recipients of their intervention. Use of these concepts will also enable students to identify stressors that may result from the conflicting demands of the various positions a person occupies simultaneously. Additionally, these concepts will enable the students to understand the distinction made between the term nurse-patient and the term nurse-client. We will begin by highlighting the concepts of position and role.

POSITION

Every person is recognized and set apart from others by a variety of titles or labels. These titles or labels designate a particular location in social space. Sarbin has indicated that society, or any aggregate of persons with a common goal, is organized or structured into positions.[1] The term position has been defined by Gouldner as the social identity that has been assigned to a person by members of his group or society.[2] Mother, wife, friend, teacher, scientist, student, and president are examples of positions in society. Thus *position* can be viewed *as the social identity assigned a particular location in social space.*

Society, furthermore, is organized in such a manner that each position has one or more complementary or counterpositions.[3] For instance, the complementary or counterpositions of daughter are daughter-mother and daughter-father. Some of the complementary or counterpositions of the nurse are: patient, doctor, aide, another nurse, hospital administrator, and social worker. Each position is differentiated with reference to one or more positions in relation to which it stands in complementary contrast.

Attached to each position are certain rights and duties.[4] The rights and obligations of a particular position are delineated in relation to the complementary counterposition. Furthermore it will be noted that the rights of one position are, in reality, the obligations of a counterposition. Sarbin defines rights as those behaviors expected of another and obligations as those behaviors directed toward others.[1] For instance, patients have the right to expect competent intervention from nurses, and nurses have the obligation to perform any nursing activities to the very best of their ability. On the other hand, nurses have the right to perform the necessary nursing procedures, and patients have the obligation to cooperate with nurses. Thus a single term such as father, doctor, nurse, or patient connotes a collection of rights and obligations as well as a location in social space.

Seldom does one stop to think about the number of positions that he or she occupies simultaneously. The reader is most likely a student, and at the same time may be a daughter or son, a wife or husband, mother or father, an employee, a sorority or fraternity member, and a friend. At this point it is suggested that the reader make a list of the positions that he or she currently occupies.

One of the many positions occupied is usually more pervasive than the others. Which is the pervasive position is often determined by such factors as money, social prestige, personal satisfactions, and life goals. Usually determination of the pervasive position is made without conscious thought, and the rights and obligations of this one position may tend to command a person's attention and govern his actions as he goes about his activities of daily living. This point will be elaborated on in a later section.

ROLE

A person assumes a position and validates his occupancy of that position by certain actions or behaviors. He enacts a role comprised of behaviors that encompass both rights and obligations. The term *role* has been defined by Turner as *that collection of behaviors thought to constitute a meaningful unit and deemed appropriate to a person occupying a particular position.*[5] In other words, a role represents what a person is supposed to do or not do in a given situation by virtue of the position that he occupies.

Who decides what is a meaningful and appropriate behavior is a logical question that might be asked. The answer evolves from an understanding of the formal and informal aspects of the role concept.*

The formal aspect of a role is comprised of those behaviors that are traditionally accepted, culturally sanctioned, or legally prescribed and are behaviors attached to or excluded from a particular position. For example, by law, registered nurses give medications to patients, but aides are not allowed to. Traditionally, fathers are not expected to take a leave of absence from their jobs to care for a newborn infant; this behavior is expected of the mother. The formal definitions of roles are learned through the socialization process, and they are based on observations of persons in various positions throughout life and are also assimilated through such avenues as reading, watching television, and formal education. The student is learning many behaviors that are meaningful and appropriate to the nurse role and is integrating them with conceptions of the nurse role held before entering the nursing program.

The second aspect of role is the informal aspect that includes those behaviors defined and agreed upon by the particular parties involved. It is a distinctly individualized matter. Cleaning house would not be listed among the formal behaviors ordinarily attached to the husband position, yet some couples are redefining their role expectations so that housecleaning is a meaningful and appropriate behavior for the husband. As interactions between two or more people evolve, they may spontaneously agree upon modifications of their roles so that their personal requirements are met.

It is essential to recognize that the definition associated with the formal aspect of any role is not static or inflexible. At one time nurses could not legally give intravenous medications, yet over a period of years this behavior has become a common practice in many critical care units. Now many state legislatures have changed their nurse practice acts so that giving intravenous medications is a formal, legally sanctioned behavior instead of being an informally accepted, although illegal, practice in a few institutions. A traditionally expected nurse behavior is that of wearing a white uniform, however, there are an increasing number of institutions in which nurses wear various colored uniforms on pediatric and medical-surgical units and street clothes on psychiatric units. It is interesting to note that these practices have not gained widespread acceptance within the profession. One can note that on the West Coast nurses tend to wear natural-colored stockings more often than not, and in the Northeast the custom of wearing white stockings is still the formally sanctioned behavior. Thus the formal aspect of role may be altered when behaviors thought to be meaningful and appropriate to a position gain widespread acceptance.

---

*The reader will find references at the end of this chapter should in-depth reading on role theory be desired.

When referring to the role of the nurse, one is speaking of the formal aspect of role in generalities with reference to those behaviors that are universally expected and accepted by the population at large. However, when one is analyzing a specific situation, both the formal and informal role aspects have to be considered. One would have to know the parties involved and their circumstances in order to assess the meaningfulness and appropriateness of the behavior in question.

There are two additional points to be made at this time about positions and roles. First, the behaviors that constitute a role for each of the many positions occupied simultaneously are not necessarily mutually exclusive. Although some behaviors are more frequently associated with one role than another, there are relatively few behaviors that are exclusively attached to only one position in our society. A man occupying the husband position may also occupy the position of a certified public accountant, and some of the behaviors of one role are also appropriate for the other. Writing checks, balancing books, preparing income tax forms are appropriate behaviors for either role. None of these three behaviors is exclusive to only one of the two positions. Feeding an infant is usually associated with a mother, but fathers, siblings, and nurses often feed young children. Although giving an injection is often thought of as an exclusive nurse behavior, under some circumstances patients and family members are taught to give injections. Prescribing narcotic medications is one example of a more exclusive behavior, since only certain kinds of doctors (laws vary from state to state) can prescribe narcotics.

On the other hand some behaviors that constitute a role are not compatible with those attached to another position occupied simultaneously. For example, a flight attendant, who is also a wife and a mother of a 2-year-old child, may find that the behavioral expectations that comprise each of her roles are not compatible. The 2-year-old requires consistency in discipline and affection; the husband desires companionship; there are the routine household chores of cooking, cleaning, washing and ironing, and marketing to be done for the family. The irregular hours, trips of 12 to 36 hours' duration, and the jet-lag fatigue problems may make the demands of the flight attendant position and of the mother, homemaker, and wife positions irreconcilable. In some cities nurses employed in municipal institutions are prohibited by law from participating in election campaigns. These nurses, who are public employees and citizens, have their ordinary citizen behaviors restricted by virtue of their particular nurse position because the law states that the municipal employees should not be involved in politics.

Beginning students in nursing should keep one final thought in mind that will encourage them during the inevitable periods of insecurity they will experience. The more practice that a person has in a given role enactment, the clearer and more differentiated the role will become. And the clearer the role is, the greater is the potential for flexibility in enactment of the role.

POSITION-ROLE: SOME PROBLEMATIC AREAS

Every human situation has its contradictions and problematic features. We will now turn our attention to some of the more ordinary problematic areas that the student will likely encounter. The authors' only intent is to create an awareness on the part of the student of some of these problematic areas, leaving an in-depth discussion to other texts where a more detailed presentation of social theory is appropriate.

Conditions and stigma* attached to the patient position-role

Society construes the patient position as an undesirable, temporary, and basically disruptive position. People do not expect to assume the patient position as a consequence of normal growth and development or as a result of ordinary activities of daily living. The position is not consciously sought by many persons in society although secondary gains of illness, especially the security of protected dependency, may lead some persons to an unconscious desire to be ill.[6] Entering the patient position usually means that a person will be thwarted in his performance of the roles with which he is normally charged. Consequently, many people refuse to assume or delay assuming the patient position because they would be hindered or actually be unable to enact the roles of other positions they occupy simultaneously. The decision to become a patient is conditioned by many factors, including the urgency of the symptoms, the previous experience with the role, and availability and accessability of health care services.

Parsons indicates that society has defined the ill person as "needing help," and as obligated to accept this help and to be cooperative with the therapeutic agent.[7] Thus to be ill is a partially and conditionally legitimized state. Parsons indicates that the essential condition of its legitimization is the recognition by the sick person that to be ill is inherently undesirable. Furthermore, the individual has an obligation to try to "get well" and to cooperate with others to this end. The person is then exempted from his normal role and task obligations in varying degrees, in varying ways, and for varying periods according to the nature of his illness.

Assuming or vacating a patient position

The nurse must understand and accept the fact that a person has the right to refuse to assume the patient position and that he also has the right to decide to vacate that position unless he constitutes a legally defined threat to other persons. Only individuals who are unable to rationally consider the consequences of their actions or who could transmit certain communicable diseases, such as tuberculosis, may

---

*The word stigma is used in a general sense. In other texts a concept of stigma will be developed with more specific implications.

be forced into or held in the patient position. There are no clear-cut guidelines that can be presented here, because the laws governing such situations are often vague and vary from state to state and city to city.

It is very difficult for a health professional to accept the fact that a person has the right to refuse formal scientific health care service, especially when he has obvious symptoms of illness. This is one of the most frustrating situations that a scientifically educated health professional will encounter. For example, people may refuse dental care when they have a toothache, may refuse to have a vision deficiency corrected by prescribed glasses, may refuse insulin injections when diagnosed as a diabetic, may refuse blood transfusions when medically indicated, may refuse medical care for broken bones, or refuse surgery that has been recommended for a cancerous condition. A variety of factors, including religious convictions, social class, or mores, to name but a few, influence a person's decision to refuse to enter or remain in the scientifically defined patient position.[8,9,10] The health professional must accept the fact that when the individual has been presented with all the possible consequences of his actions, unless there is a legally defined health threat consideration, his professional obligations have been fulfilled, even though his recommendations may not be followed.

Learning a new role

A person assuming a new position has some general notions about the behaviors that are a logical part of the new role. However, it takes time to refine and clarify the totality of behavioral expectations appropriate and meaningful to the new role whether it be assuming the position of committee chairman, a college student, or a nurse. There is an adjustment period during which the role is discerned and solidified in the person's mind.

One natural tendency when assuming a new position is to look for absolutes or things that should or should not be done. This is a "cookbook" approach in contrast to the "haute cuisine" approach. One is based on a specific recipe (ingredients, amounts, and time all prespecified) while the other is based on principles, on knowing what combinations of ingredients will achieve the desired results. The cook using the latter method is not limited to a book of recipes but can create new dishes with ingredients on hand.

In some positions the "cookbook" approach is useful, such as in the in-service training of aides; however, it is too limiting for the nurse position. Although do's and don'ts may be helpful at the time, they do not prepare the student for the future. The "do and don't" approach leads to rigidity in role enactment because the person does not learn how to assess and judge the situation for himself. He develops a dependency on rules and regulations to govern his actions and interactions. To make this point more meaningful, we will use the student situation to illustrate the problem.

A faculty member can anticipate that sooner or later the following questions will arise in every group of students interacting with clients either in the hospital or community setting:

1. Is it all right to call the patient by his first name or have the patient call me by mine?
2. May I give the patient a ride home from the clinic if it is convenient for me to do so?
3. May I run an errand for the patient who is confined to the hospital or home?
4. Should I accept coffee or food from the family when I am making a home visit?
5. May I give the patient money or should I accept money from the patient?

The above questions about behaviors of a nurse indicate that the student is unsure of whether the behavior is compatible in the nurse position. Limiting the discussion to the "name calling" question for illustration, the students should be encouraged to ask themselves the following questions rather than accepting a direct yes or no answer:

1. In our society and in this section of the country, what is the meaning of the use of first names or of titles?
2. What is the structural variable profile of the other person and of myself?
3. What are the possible positive and negative outcomes that might be predicted?
4. Whose needs am I actually meeting? The patient's or my own?

Thinking through the answers to such questions with a faculty member will strengthen the student's ability to cope with other situations when questions about appropriate behavior arise.

From the answers to the above questions it can be seen that calling or being called by the first name is not incompatible with the nurse position, provided that the nurse is secure in the enactment of the other nurse role behaviors. Under some circumstances calling or being called by the first name may have positive outcomes that outweigh any negative ones. Other times the reverse may be true. Experienced nurses may call or be called by their first names without role confusion. However, their choice is based on the prediction of positive outcomes for the patient. It is hoped that this brief highlighting of one simple situation will encourage the students to problem solve other situations of a similar nature and that it will become an inherent part of their thought process rather than developing the tendency to depend entirely upon a set of externally imposed rules and regulations.

Emphasis on rights and obligations

The rights and obligations attached to a position are two sides of the same coin and cannot be disassociated. For some reason, perhaps because of the life-threatening circumstances in the health field, the emphasis tends to be placed on the obligations of the positions. Too often the rights of a position are deemphasized. Rights of the patient position as well as the rights of the nurse are ignored or violated too frequently.

The patient, for instance, has the right to expect to be treated as a person and not as an object occupying a bed. He has the right to be informed about what is happening to him and around him. Violations of this right have led to the introduction of *informed consent*. The patient must be given *all* the information (in language that is understandable) upon which to make a decision about a particular procedure or course of action. This means inclusion of both the possible positive and negative outcomes if he agrees with the actions as well as the possible positive and negative outcomes if he should oppose the action. One of the appropriate behaviors of the nurse role that has been formally acknowledged only in the past few years is that of "patient advocate." Often the patient is either uninformed about his rights or too ill to do anything about the situation. A nurse or nurses can intervene on behalf of a patient or group of patients when it is recognized that the patient's rights are not being fulfilled or are actually being violated. It is interesting to note that in some states, patient advocacy groups (general public and health professionals) have been able to get the state legislators to adopt a "Patient's Bill of Rights" law. Some hospitals voluntarily provide their patients with a bill of rights form because in actual practice patient rights had not previously been fully acknowledged.

It is safe to say that nurses have always been concerned about their obligations to the patient; however, only in recent years have nurses begun to be more vocal about their rights as nurses. Some still find it difficult to accept the fact that unless rights are acknowledged, fulfillment of their obligations is impaired. For example, nurses have the right to expect adequate supplies with which to work available in both quantity and quality. They have the right to expect adequate pay, staffing patterns, and to have available prompt medical support when it is needed. Of course, nurses, too, have the right to expect to be treated as respected and capable persons by both patients and by other staff members.

You must keep in mind that rights and obligations constitute an inseparable and delicately balanced unit. As indicated on p. 104 rights are those behaviors expected of others and obligations are those behaviors directed toward others. A role can be productively enacted only if both the rights and the obligations of a position are clearly defined and accepted by all those concerned.

Delegation of role behaviors

It was stated on p. 104 that there are specific rights and obligations attached to every position, which are fulfilled by certain behaviors. The area of knowledge and skills necessary as a basis for fulfillment of the nurse's rights and obligations (professional nursing practice) has been defined by the profession. Nurses are legally and morally responsible for performing competently within this framework.

Nurses must recognize that even though they may delegate a particular act or behavior to another person, the responsibility for its outcomes cannot be delegated. The nurse remains accountable for its consequences. For example, if the nurse assigns an aide the task of bathing a patient, the nurse is responsible for all that occurs. Therefore, nurses must evaluate the situation carefully to ensure that their professional responsibilities will be fulfilled by the actions of another person.

Because of the daily pressures in nursing, nurses are prone to consider an activity as an end in and of itself (Chapter 7) and delegate indiscriminately to other categories of health workers. To avoid this compromising situation, the nurse must keep in mind that the delegation process includes four steps:

1. Assessment of the needs of the patient
2. Identification of the expected outcomes of the specific activity to be delegated
3. Assessment of the capabilities of the person to whom the activity is to be delegated
4. Evaluation of the total situation when the delegated activity is completed

It must be added that nursing personnel are notorious for possessiveness of what they perceive as their role. Nurses are often very reluctant to relinquish behaviors to people outside the nursing staff, even though the nonnursing person may handle them well. This attitude can be a stressor for the nurse, patient, and his family. The idea of a family member giving a patient a bath while he is in the hospital can be very disturbing to the nurse. Some nurses view it as a infringement into their territorial rights without assessing the advantages and disadvantages to the patient. There are times when the patient's family members, as well as the patient, could benefit from an interactional activity, even though the task might not be done quite as proficiently. Recently a woman was encouraged to help with the feeding of her husband while he was immobilized in the hospital. The husband appreciated being fed by his wife because he could eat the food while it was hot and not be rushed through his meal, and the wife appreciated it because it eased her sense of helplessness. It is hoped that the nurse will be willing to assess the specific situation and to delegate certain behaviors to family members or "significant others" when it is beneficial to all involved.

It is essential to examine the situation existing when activities are delegated to the nurse. Nurses carry out many tasks on behalf of professionals from other disciplines who have knowledge and skills differing from those of the nurse. Nurses perform many activities that are delegated to them by doctors for which the doctor retains responsibility for the consequences.

There are nursing judgments to be made before performing any delegated activity. The very decision to perform a delegated procedure or task is a critical nursing judgment. Nurses should not indiscriminately do something just because it has been ordered by a doctor. There are two conditions under which nurses should refuse to accept delegations:

1. If the nurse knows that it is beyond his or her own capabilities, even though another nurse may be able to perform the task or its performance would be expected of nurses in general.
2. If, based on the body of knowledge and skills for which the nurse is held professionally accountable, he or she has reason to question the judgment of the doctor's order in the particular situation.

If the nurse does undertake a delegated activity under either of the above conditions, he or she would be legally and professionally responsible for any negative outcomes. Of course under the latter condition, the doctor as well as the nurse could be held legally accountable. Most important, nurses can often prevent adverse consequences for the patient as well as themselves and the doctors when they are judicious about accepting responsibility for such activities as might be delegated to them.

Occasionally doctors and staff nurses will inadvertently put a student into a situation for which he or she is not yet prepared without the awareness of the supervising faculty member. It is often difficult for a student to say no to a request or an order from a doctor or staff nurse. However, students can be helped to face this dilemma in the classroom by role playing a variety of responses that could appropriately be made in order to exempt themselves from a responsibility for which they are unprepared.

Role confusion

On p. 104 the point was made that a person is always occupying several positions simultaneously, and on p. 106 the point was made that many behaviors comprising the various roles are not mutually exclusive. Because some of the behaviors of the various roles are not mutually exclusive, identification of which role is being enacted may be unclear to the parties involved. Obviously the behavioral expectations will vary greatly depending upon which position is identified as dominant or governing in the situation.

The student should be aware that occasionally a patient will not be certain whether he should respond to the student as a student, as a nurse, as a son or daughter, or as a friend. For instance, a student may be very solicitous or protective of a patient, appropriate under the specific circumstances; however, the patient may respond to this solicitous or protective behavior inappropriately as a friend or parent to the student. In some cases the dominant position governing the interaction may be unclear in the patient's mind, either in fact or because he wishes another position to be dominant.

Conversely, the nurse may not be sure which role of the various positions that the patient occupies is being enacted. For example, a patient asks the nurse her first name and details about her personal life. Is he doing this so that he will feel more comfortable in the patient position, or are these the first behaviors apparent in the enactment of the friend or boyfriend role?

Validation of role enactment must sometimes be made directly and immediately in order to avoid confusion, which is a potential stressor to both the nurse and the patient. There are times when a person will recognize the need to indicate which position he is enacting may do so by saying: "I am your nurse," or "speaking as your nurse," or "speaking as your attorney." Similarly, confirmation of the role another person is enacting can usually be gained by simply asking, "Are you speaking as my lawyer or asking as a friend?" Of course, throughout the nursing program the student will be learning many other techniques useful in these situations.

It should be emphasized that nurses themselves will sometimes be unaware that they have shifted roles during a given interaction. One rather classic situation occurred when a student became upset and angry because a patient related to her as a girl friend. He attempted to hold her hand and asked her for a date. In a follow-up conference, the student's classmates pointed out a variety of seductive behaviors that they had observed on the part of the student. They pointed out the winking, the physical closeness whenever talking to the patient, the fact that the top two buttons of her uniform were always unbuttoned, and so on. The student was unaware that her own behavior had encouraged the patient to see her more prominently as a female–girl friend than as a nurse. After role playing a "corrective interaction" with her classmates, the student returned to the patient. She related her discomfort with his behavior, indicated that she may have unconsciously given him cues that could be misinterpreted, and discussed her position and role as a student in nursing. After this episode, they were able to continue with an amicable nurse-patient relationship.

On p. 106 the point was made that some behaviors that comprise a role are not compatible with those of other positions. Thus the conflicting demands of the various positions occupied may be a stressor for the person. For instance, in order to fulfill the behavioral expectations for the student position, the behaviors associated with other positions occupied sometimes have to be deemphasized or omitted. The student may have less time to date, to do housework, or to handle a job. Sometimes adjustments can be made without intensification of the stress state, but other times the conflicting demands can lead to a very precarious behavioral stability.

The person who becomes a patient may give priority to this position, yet feel very guilty about not fulfilling his normal daily obligations. Nurses can help to make the patient position more tolerable and reduce the stress intensification by reinforcing the legitimacy of the patient role. People often need to be reminded that illness exempts them from their usual positional obligations and roles (p. 107); this fact seems so obvious that it is often overlooked. However, what an individual defines as "being sick" (Chapter 5) determines both what he views as legitimate and the ease with which he can accept the patient position.

The nurse who is alert to the many positions that the patient occupies frequently can be instrumental in easing the tension that can occur when the person is unable to fulfill his other obligations. For example, the nurse might be a catalyst in: (1) notification of the employer so that an official medical leave could be instituted, or (2) soliciting the assistance of family members or significant others to fulfill some of the other position obligations, such as child or pet care, on a temporary basis, or (3) encouraging the college student with a fractured femur to have other students come in to tutor him so that he can keep up with the class material. When nurses are aware of some of the role conflicts, there are innumerable ways in which they can assist the person so that he may be more comfortable in his position as a patient.

Sometimes the decision of position priority and role enactment at a given point in time may be inappropriate. A female college student may be more concerned about becoming a wife than a nurse. Consequently she may enact more behaviors appropriate to the girl friend position than the student position while she is in the college library. A priest who was involved in a car accident was admitted to the hospital with head injuries. Several hours later the nurse and the hospital chaplain found the priest across the hall giving last rites to a dying patient. Although the priest's intentions were good, his role enactment was very inappropriate under the circumstances.

Still other times, the position that is pervasive or most central in a person's life will be enacted throughout his waking hours, making enactment of more appropriate positions-roles virtually impossible. A man sometimes referred to as a "workaholic" may eat, dream, and socialize his business responsibilities to the exclusion of anything more than a token acknowledgment of his husband, son, father, or friend positions. A nurse may be observed enacting her professional role with her children and other relatives, with friends, or even strangers; this can occur at home, at social outings, or in passing on the street, and the help may be neither requested or needed. The inability to appropriately enact the various roles is a maladaptive behavior; its causes and the interventions are discussed in depth in other texts.

There is one last problematic area to be acknowledged in this discussion. Unfortunately, sometimes nurses relate to a person's pervasive position rather than the appropriate counterposition of patient. This can occur, for example, when a patient occupies either a high- or low-prestige position. In either of these cases the nursing judgment may be modified or skewed because of another position that the person occupies simultaneously. If the person admitted to a hospital is a senator, a doctor, or a well-known actor (high-prestige positions), deference may be shown to him that is not usually accorded to other patients. For instance, certain routine patient care procedures may be altered, such as not awakening the well-known actor with the rest of the patients for a "pre-seven AM wash-up." Although many of the other patients may have the need for additional sleep, only the actor is allowed the extra sleep time. Conversely, sometimes the health care needs of high-prestige patients are ignored. One hospital still has a rule that all individuals on a unit reserved for wealthy or renowned people are to be given a bed bath daily. The bed bath is considered a service for which the person is paying, and even though it might be more advantageous for a particular person's recuperation to have him assist with or actually take his own bath, it is "forbidden." In the case of a low-prestige position such as that of a skid-row bum or drug addict, the nurse may make noticeably fewer trips into their rooms and respond more slowly to their call bells. There are many little ways in which discrimination can be manifested if the nurse relates to the pervasive low-prestige position. All patients, regardless of what other positions are occupied concurrently, deserve the highest quality care that it is possible for the nurse to give. The nurse must be careful that because of her own value system, care is not biased by other positions the patient occupies simultaneously.

This concludes the highlighting of some of the common problematic areas you will encounter in the student and nurse positions. We will now turn our attention to the confusion that clouds the terms of nurse-patient and nurse-client.

MAJOR COUNTERPOSITION FOR THE NURSE

You will find frequent references to "nurse-patient interactions" or "nurse-patient relationships" in the literature; however, only occasionally will you find reference to a "nurse-client relationship." The term nurse-client is a more inclusive term and its usage is becoming more prevalent; therefore, we will discuss the distinction made between the term "client" and "patient," and set forth the reasons for the increasing acceptance of the term client in all settings.

The debate often centers around the question, "At what point does a person enter the patient position?" Some will say that a person enters the patient position when he has signs or symptoms of some sort of pathologic condition, while others will argue that it is at the point when a person places himself under medical care for those signs and symptoms. A patient is literally defined as a person who is under medical or surgical treatment.[11] The attempt to broaden the definition of the term patient is, itself, symptomatic of a problem. However, debating the point at which a person enters the patient position does nothing to clarify the real issue at hand.

The real issue is whether or not the term patient encompasses all people who utilize nursing service, or, more precisely, health care service. The issue comes into focus when one recognizes that health service has four dimensions: (1) preven-

tion, (2) early detection, (3) treatment during illness, and (4) rehabilitation following the resolution of a pathologic condition. These four dimensions occur in every
setting in which nurses practice; however, the degree of emphasis on each of the
four dimensions will vary from setting to setting. The delivery of health service
would be restricted to the illness dimension if health care were actually limited to
those who are patients. There is a role for the nurse in interactions with people that
is negated by limiting the nurse to a nurse-patient relationship. Consequently, because of the restrictive nature of the term patient that surfaces when one considers
the four dimensions of health care, use of the term client has evolved.

A client can be defined as a person who seeks the specialized assistance of another, a consumer. A client in the health care field is one who, regardless of his
place on the health continuum, can be assisted to attain or maintain the highest possible level of wellness (Chapter 5). Clients may be patients; clients may be persons
who have been patients but who can attain a higher level of wellness when assisted
to adjust their activities of daily living to most constructively accommodate their
residual disabilities; clients may be people who have the potential for becoming
patients unless they alter some maladaptive behavior of daily living; clients may
be people who have a high level of wellness yet who can utilize assistance to maintain that level. The distinction made between the terms client and patient is based
on the inclusion of the four dimensions of health care in nursing practice and the
subsequent determination of what persons are candidates for the nurse's service.
Some of the more specific arguments supporting the use of the inclusive term client
are highlighted in the following three paragraphs.

Many nurses work in areas where the focus is primarily preventive rather than
restorative, and these nurses frequently do not have a nurse-patient relationship by
standard definition. Nurses working in health departments, industry, schools, and
a variety of other community agencies often work with people who do not have
signs or symptoms of illness or who are not under the care of a physician. Sometimes they are working with individuals who have a lowered level of wellness that
can be attributed to maladaptive behaviors of daily living, with a potential for pathologic conditions developing unless they can be motivated to alter some of their daily
living patterns. One example would be a teenager whose diet consists of what are
commonly called "junk foods." Sometimes these nurses work with people who
have a high level of wellness and the nursing intervention assists them to maintain
that level. For instance, nurses may have many interactions with people intended
to raise the level of "conscious awareness" about routine screening procedures for
early detection, about healthy life-styles and good health habits, and about environmental conditions essential in order to maintain or attain a yet higher level of wellness. Of course, other times nurses in community settings do work with people
who are patients in the literal sense of the word. However, the term client fits the

scope of nursing practice in the community setting more accurately than does the term patient.

The doctor-nurse-patient triad is the traditional way of viewing the delivery of health care. Some nurses will argue that their function within this triad tends to be viewed as the "handmaiden of the physician," which in turn limits their ability to use the full scope of their own nursing knowledge and skills when interacting with the health care consumer. These nurses believe that the term client reinforces the idea of a contractual agreement between nurses and care recipients for the contribution of their autonomous nursing judgments that are complementary and supplementary to those of the physician. Moreover, many nurses also prefer the term client because the word patient is associated with illness, which, they believe, reinforces the dichotomy between health and illness; focusing attention on levels of wellness broadens the scope of practice to include the four dimensions of health care regardless of the setting.

Some nurses also support the usage of the term client because it has the connotation of active participation on the part of the health care recipient. The patient role as defined by Parsons is a dependent position-role.[7] Many nurses have erroneously equated a dependent position with a passive participation on the part of the patient. An analogous situation is that of a 4-year-old child. This position, too, is a dependent position, but if the child is to grow and learn from his experiences, he must be considered an active participant in the process. For example, the child learns from attempting to tie his shoelaces, not from continually having them tied for him. A similar situation exists for the person who is hospitalized; like some parents, some nurses encourage dependency in unwarranted situations, which denies the person appropriate learning experiences during his illness. Consequently, some nurses use the term client because it reinforces the idea that the care recipient actively participates in the process even though he occupies a dependent position.

Although the impetus for using the term client may vary from setting to setting, the main focus of the movement is the same. *Nurses, collectively, are concerned about incorporating the four dimensions of health care into their practice and are considering the consumer of their service as a person who can be actively engaged, regardless of where he is on the health continuum, in attaining or maintaining the highest possible level of wellness.* The position of client, when counter to that of the nurse, includes all people who utilize the services of a nurse to attain or maintain the highest possible level of wellness; therefore, the term client is the most legitimate term because it is the more inclusive complementary counterposition for the nurse.

Unfortunately, the position of client does not automatically symbolize a relationship in the health care field as graphically or as exclusively as does the position of patient. There are many different positions that have client as a complementary counterposition; attorney, stockbroker, real estate agent all have client as a counterposition. It is probably for this reason that many nurses still habitually use the word patient in situations in which the term client is more accurate. However, the discussion of the nurse-client relationship in the next chapter should resolve any lingering concerns that might be generated when the term client is used.

SUMMARY

The interrelated concepts of position and of role have been used to provide the nurse with another dimension in analysis of behavioral expectations and potential stressors in a variety of social settings and under differing conditions. To reiterate, position is defined as the social identity assigned a particular location in social space, and role is defined as that collection of behaviors thought to constitute a meaningful unit and deemed appropriate to a person occupying a particular position. A role comprises behaviors that encompass both rights and obligations. The traditionally accepted, culturally sanctioned, or legally prescribed behaviors attached to or excluded from a particular position constitute the formal aspect of a role. It was pointed out that the formal aspect of role is not a static definition of behaviors but changes when there is widespread acceptance by the population at large. Every role has an informal aspect that includes those behaviors defined and agreed upon by the particular parties involved to meet the requirements of their special circumstances.

Since nursing involves an interactional process, the behavioral stability of both the nurse and the client is a reciprocal factor; the behavioral stability of all the interactional participants can be affected by role confusion as well as the conflicting demands of the rights and obligations attached to the various positions occupied simultaneously by any individual. These stressors need to be identified so that appropriate action can be undertaken. The answers to the following questions will help to identify potential stressors in the situation and give direction to nursing intervention:

1. What does the person view as his rights and obligations in the client position?
2. What is his understanding of the client role and the role of the nurse? Are they the same as the understandings of the nurse?
3. What other positions does he occupy simultaneously? Is one of them more dominant than the others?
4. Can confusion or conflict between the roles attached to his other positions and the client role be anticipated?
5. Are there any cues that indicate how rigid or flexible the person is in enactment of his various roles?

Additionally, nurses must ask themselves the following questions at frequent intervals, since their actions both influence and are affected by the client's behavior:

1. Am I fulfilling the full scope of my professional obligations in my daily practice?
2. Are my rights as a professional nurse being acknowledged in such a way that I can best fulfill my professional obligations?
3. To what degree am I depending upon external rules and regulations to govern my actions?
4. Is there role rigidity setting in my interactions with clients?
5. Are my professional obligations being fulfilled when I delegate some tasks to other categories of health workers or family members?
6. Am I accepting responsibility judiciously for tasks delegated to me?
7. Do I shift roles inadvertently when the nurse position is the governing position?
8. Are there conflicting demands of other positions I occupy that influence my enactment of the nurse role?

Enactment of the nurse role will be more effective when nurses incorporate this line of questioning into their assessment process.

Finally, it was indicated that although either the patient or the client position is a legitimate counterposition for the nurse, the more inclusive client position is the most legitimate position. The term client is used more frequently in the community settings; however, it is gaining support within hospitals. A client is a person who may be actively engaged, regardless of where he is on the health continuum, in attaining or maintaining a high level of wellness. Arguments supporting usage of the term client can be summarized as follows: the term client (1) includes all people who utilize the service of a nurse to maintain or attain a higher level of wellness, (2) reinforces the inclusion of the four dimensions of health care that should be included in varying degrees in all settings, (3) deemphasizes the dichotomy between health and illness, which is reinforced by the term patient that is associated with illness, (4) reinforces the area of nursing's autonomous contribution to health care as complemental and supplemental to that of the physician, and (5) connotes an active participation on the part of the recipient.

The next chapter will deal with the nature of the relationship that exists between the nurse and the nursing care recipient, who throughout the chapter will be referred to as a client.

REFERENCES

1. Sarbin, T. R.: Role theory. In Lindzey, G., editor: Handbook of social psychology, ed. 2, vol. 1, Reading, Mass., 1954, Addison-Wesley Publishing Co., Inc., pp. 223-244.
2. Gouldner, A. W.: Cosmopolitan and locals: towards an analysis of latent social roles, I, Administration Science Quarterly **2:**281-306, 1957.

3. Hunt, R. G.: Role and role conflict. In Hollander, E. P., and Hunt, R. G., editors: Current perspectives in social psychology, New York, 1971, Oxford University Press, pp. 279-285.
4. Levinson, Daniel J.: Role, personality and social structure in the organizational setting, Journal of Abnormal and Social Psychology **58:**170-180, 1959.
5. Turner, Ralph H.: Role taking, role standpoint and reference group behavior, American Journal of Sociology **61:**316-328, 1956.
6. Wilson, Robert N.: Patient-practitioner relationship. In Reeder, L. G., editor: Handbook of Medical Sociology, Englewood Cliffs, N.J., 1963, Prentice-Hall, Inc., pp. 273-295.
7. Parsons, Talcott: The social system, New York, 1951, The Free Press, pp. 428-473.
8. King, S. H.: System of beliefs and attitudes about disease, perceptions of illness and medical practice, New York, 1962, Russell Sage Foundation, pp. 91-97.
9. Wardwell, W. I.: Limited, marginal and quasi-practitioners. In Reeder, L. G., editor: Handbook of medical sociology, Englewood Cliffs, N.J., 1963, Prentice-Hall, Inc., pp. 224-235.
10. Jaco, E. G.: Socio-cultural aspects of medical care and treatment, patients, physicians and illness, New York, 1963, The Free Press, pp. 181-245.
11. Stein, Jess, editor: The Random House dictionary of the English language, unabridged edition, New York, 1966, Random House, Inc.

ADDITIONAL READINGS

Bandman, Elsie, and Bandman, Bertram: There is nothing automatic about rights, American Journal of Nursing **77:**867-872, 1977.
Biddle, Bruce, and Thomas, Edwin: Role theory: concepts and research, New York, 1966, John Wiley & Sons, Inc.
Goode, W. J.: A theory of role strain, American Sociological Review **25:**403-496, 1960.
Katz, Daniel, and Kahn, Robert: The social psychology of organizations, New York, 1966, John Wiley & Sons, Inc., Chap. 7.
Kramer, Marlene: Reality shock, St. Louis, 1974, The C. V. Mosby Co.
Lawless, David: Effective management: social psychology approaches, Englewood Cliffs, N.J., 1972, Prentice-Hall, Inc., Chap. 15.
Levine, Myra E.: Nursing ethics and the ethical nurse, American Journal of Nursing **77:**845-848, 1977.
Moore, Wilbur: The professional, rules and roles, New York, 1970, Russell Sage Foundation.

Chapter 9

THE NURSE-CLIENT RELATIONSHIP

Chapter 8 indicated that designation of a position-role and a complementary counterposition-role delineates the specific nature of the relationship that should ensue. The effectiveness of nurse-client interactions can be maximized when from its onset the nature of the relationship is clear in the minds of the participants and when the nurse incorporates all the stages of a relationship during the interactional process. However, in order to examine the specific nature of the nurse-client relationship, it is necessary, first, to understand the concept of a relationship. This chapter will be devoted to an examination of a relationship concept and its implications for the nurse-client relationship.

A RELATIONSHIP CONCEPT

A *relationship* can be defined as a *goal-directed interaction between two people or collection of individuals that is mutually determined and accepted.* All relationships do consist of interactions, but not all interactions constitute a relationship. For instance, a person may nod his head or say "Good morning" to another person in passing; he may offer his seat on the bus to another; or may ask someone if he knows the price of an item in a store. These are interactions between people but are not necessarily relationships. If the persons were to continue their conversation, a mutual interest might be identified and they might agree to continue their interactions, thereby establishing a relationship. Perhaps in the aforementioned interaction between the two people on the bus, casual conversation was continued and when they discovered a common interest in classical music, they made plans to attend a concert together the following week. Their interaction culminated in a social relationship.

This chapter was developed and prepared in collaboration with Mary Ann Preach, R.N., M.S., Professor, El Camino College, Torrance, California.

Agreement to interact

All relationships are based upon some sort of a "contract" between those involved. Seldom do we think of a relationship as constituted by a contract between individuals; however, in actuality it is. Children put things so simply: "I'll be your friend if you will be my friend." If one or the other is not satisfied with the bargain, he will vacate the friend position with the other person, thereby dissolving their relationship. There is a more formal agreement between an employer and employee. If an employee feels that his rights are being violated or if he is unwilling to assume the obligations attached to his position, he may resign or be fired. Thus for a relationship to exist, there is a stated or implied contract of some sort, and that relationship may be dissolved when either party is unwilling to abide by the stated or implied agreement. It is therefore important for us to examine more specifically just what should be included in the relationship agreement.

Components of a relationship agreement

Any bargain, pact, or contract includes the following four basic components, which are universal components of every relationship.

1. *Goals*. This is the specification of the purpose and objectives for the relationship. Both parties must agree on what is to be achieved through their interactions.
2. *Benefits*. There must be an understanding of how any gains, profits, advantages, or assistance will be apportioned to each of the participants in the relationship.
3. *Duration*. It is important that the participants have a tentative and a realistic expectation of their time involvement. They must have some understanding about the length of time to be committed to achieve the goals. Duration may have a more or less specific time allotment or may be open-ended in nature.
4. *Conditions*. The participants need to understand what, if any, conditions or constraints are attached to the relationship. They need to know what areas cannot be violated or what actions would void the contract or place the relationship in jeopardy.

People rarely spend much time considering the components that provide the ground rules for their relationship. Too often each participant has his own conception of the specific nature of these components and assumes that the other person has the same ideas that he has. Thus, the majority of relationships involve a loose commitment that is very general or unspecific in nature; and, until a dispute arises, this vagueness may be acceptable. Since the majority of the general public does not conceive of a relationship as a contract or agreement with specific negotiable items and conditions, the nurse may need to take the lead to ensure that the ground rules of the nurse-client relationship are explicitly agreed upon rather than taken for granted.

The implications of this statement will become more apparent when the nurse-client relationship is discussed.

•　　•　　•

When examining the concept of a relationship one would ordinarily, at this point, discuss the three stages that should occur in any relationship. We believe, however, that the three stages will have more meaning for you if they are discussed within the framework of the nurse-client relationship so that the general points can be illustrated with nursing examples. Therefore we have elected to postpone discussion of the stages until after the nurse-client relationship has been developed.

NURSE-CLIENT RELATIONSHIPS

An individual throughout his lifetime will engage in many different types of relationships; however, we will focus our attention on only one type, that type existing when a nurse and a client interact. As a nurse moves from peripheral social space into a position of professional significance to a particular person or group of individuals, he or she assumes the position of an assisting or helping person. The person accepting the help assumes the client position. This *nurse-client relationship is defined as a professional relationship that occurs when the nurse and another person have entered into an agreement to interact to achieve some mutually determined health-oriented goals that are consistent with nursing's professional obligations.*

Some kinds of relationships are informal in nature, while other types are highly formalized. The professional relationship, which is formalized, has five unique characteristics that must be considered: (1) one person must have knowledge and skills from which another can benefit; (2) the needs or requirements of the person to be assisted must take priority over those of the helping person; (3) the relationship is self-limiting by virtue of the goals to be achieved; (4) the person to be helped must want and utilize the assistance; and (5) the assistance must be given competently. The specific nature of the nurse-client relationship will become apparent when the five characteristics of a professional relationship are correlated in the following sections with the four basic components of any relationship agreement.

Goals

In association with the word nurse, the term *health-oriented goals* has a very specific meaning for the following reasons. In the general scheme of things, society has assigned to *all* health professionals the responsibility of helping to ensure that individuals can achieve the highest possible level of wellness within the limitations of their situations. (It must be remembered that health professionals is a broad term that includes dentists, dieticians, physicians, psychologists, nurses, and physical therapists, to name but a few.) Furthermore, society, under this broad umbrella, has assigned more specific obligations to each of the many complementary counter-positions of the various health professionals. These obligations are statements utilized for the division of labor and general coordination of activities among the various disciplines. For example, society has assigned the responsibility of diagnosing and prescribing treatments to prevent or cure psychophysiopathologic conditions to the complementary position of physician. *Society has assigned the nurse the responsibility for assisting the client, as a unified whole, to adjust his activities of daily living so that his steady state is maintained or regained while he is moving to a higher level of wellness.* Thus the health-oriented goals are delineated by the nurse's professional obligations that are determined by society. The specific nature of the health objectives will vary, of course, depending upon where the individual is on the wellness continuum.

It is not surprising to find many gray areas between the counterpositions of the various health professionals both because their obligations are complementary and collaborative in nature and because the formal definition of any role does not remain static. Throughout their careers, nurses must continue to discern the most current delineation between behaviors that they should initiate based on their own body of knowledge and skills and those behaviors that are undertaken only at the direction of various other health professionals.

Benefits

Inherent in a professional type of relationship is the fact that *the health needs of the client take precedence over the personal needs of the nurse as he or she enacts the nurse role.* Obviously this means that the nurse's role must be enacted in such a way that the client will benefit from the interactions; the client must receive the required nursing assistance. There most certainly can and should be benefits to the nurse occurring coincidentally. Nurses earn a salary for enacting the nurse role. Moreover, nurses can learn from their clients, can enjoy their company, and can garner a great many satisfactions from being a catalyst in their client's progress. However, at such times when there is a conflict between the health needs of the client and the personal needs of the nurse, the client's needs always take precedence.

It is unrealistic to expect nurses to totally subordinate their own personal needs in all client situations. Because the benefits to the nurse are secondary to those of the client, there will be times when a nurse must admit that he or she cannot work effectively with a particular client. Nurses cannot be all things to all people; those nurses who attempt this either will, unknowingly, be ineffective with some clients or may be effective at great cost to their own behavioral stability.

Duration

The duration of a nurse-client relationship is temporary and is directly related to the health goals to be achieved. There are no set criteria upon which the time span of a relationship can be based. A relationship may be long term if the client requires a great amount of assistance and if the client would be placed in precarious stability if the assistance were given too rapidly. Examples include: the one-to-one therapy in long-term psychiatric rehabilitation; the relationship the public health nurse has with a multigenerational and multiproblem family; and the oncology nurse's relationship with the patient who has cancer. These relationships may extend for months or even years rather than days or weeks. On the other hand, the nurse-client relationship may be short term because the health goals do not warrant an extended time period for achievement. As an example, the relationship with a person who has a high level of wellness but suddenly requires an appendectomy may exist for only a matter of days.

Discussion of a time reference can help to minimize stress intensification in different ways. Parkinson's law states that work expands to the time allowed.[1] If a reasonable time limit is not established, either the nurse or the client may waste valuable time by presuming there is an indefinite period to achieve the goals. By stating the time dimension, the work of accomplishing the goals can then be apportioned realistically.

The nurse must often assist the client in determining whether the goals are realistic in terms of the duration. Some clients may become disturbed with the apparent slowness of their progress if they have unrealistic expectations of what can be accomplished in a given period of time. For example, a person may expect to resume most of his ordinary activities 2 or 3 days after major surgery. The nurse who immediately identifies a client's unrealistic expectations can reinforce, from the onset of the relationship, a more accurate time dimension for the resumption of ordinary activities.

The relationship may seem too short if the secondary gains of the client position become paramount. Companionship, for instance, is an acceptable concomitant benefit, but it is not a valid reason for continuing the relationship when the established health-related goals have been achieved. The nurse can forestall this development by reinforcing the time frame's correlation with the established health objectives. This action will help keep the client's attention focused upon the central objectives of the relationship, which are the determining factors for its continuance.

Some people may be concerned that their relationship with a nurse may have an arbitrary cutoff point unrelated to their demonstrated needs. Discussion of the anticipated duration of the relationship can be reassuring to a client when he understands that assistance and resources will be available to him until the mutually determined goals have been achieved. In each of these situations, background knowledge of patterns of behavior, of the automatic regulatory processes, and experiences with a wide variety of health problems will enable the nurse to help the client in understanding and adjusting to the expected course of events in his particular situation. Moreover, termination of a relationship will seem less abrupt if the time frame has been discussed at the onset of the relationship.

Conditions

The conditions imposed on the nurse-client relationship evolve from the rights and obligations attached to each of the complementary counterpositions of nurse and of client. Obviously the nurse will consider all the rights and obligations that impose constraints of some sort on his or her nurse-client relationship. However, our discussion will be limited to the conditions of foremost importance to any nurse-client relationship.

First, the nurse must competently give the assistance essential to the welfare of the client. If the nurse's performance does not meet the patient's needs, or if professional practice standards are not maintained, the client may refuse that nurse's assistance.

Second, the client must want to achieve a higher level of wellness and must cooperate with the nurse to the best of his ability. A person who has obvious symptoms of illness may be very willing or even eager to accept this condition of the nurse-client relationship. If a person is operating at a low level of wellness but without any recognized pathologic condition, he is more apt to violate the above condition, which places the relationship in jeopardy. Some individuals, particularly in the community setting, may not realize the advantages of a nurse-client relationship. For this reason some nurse-client interactions do not culminate in a relationship, because the person who could be helped does not see or accept the need for assistance. At other times a relationship may be initiated, but it becomes evident that the person is unwilling to appropriately enact the client role. Since the client does not assume the obligations, the conditions are violated and the relationship is abrogated.

NURSING STUDENT–CLIENT RELATIONSHIPS

Students in nursing programs are acquiring knowledge and skills that will enable them to enact the role of the nurse, and they are often confused about the nature of their relationship with the client during this period. For this reason it is important to identify the differences between the student-client and the nurse-client relationships. A nursing student–client relationship differs from that of a nurse-client relationship in the following respects:

1. *Goals.* In this situation there are two overlapping sets of goals and objectives: the usual health-oriented objectives of the client and the educational objectives of the student.

2. *Benefits.* Both the client and the student must benefit simultaneously from their interactions. However, the client's health needs will take precedence over the educational needs of the student should a conflict arise.

3. *Duration.* The time factor is governed by the time it takes to achieve the educational goals of the student rather than the time necessary to achieve the health goals of the client.

4. *Conditions.* The competency expectations of the student are based on the knowledge and skills that he or she has acquired up to that point in the educational process. It is expected that the student will perform any assignment safely, but the degree of proficiency may vary widely. As the student approaches completion of the educational program, the performance expectations will near the competency standards expected of the beginning nurse practitioner.

It is the responsibility of the faculty members to ensure that clinical experiences are selected that will enable both the client and the student to achieve their goals during the nursing student–client relationship. However, when students understand the nature of their relationship with the client, they will be in a better position to maximize the learning experiences afforded them and to be more effective with the client.

We have indicated that when the complementary counterpositions are designated as nurse-client, the resulting relationship is a professional type of relationship. The special characteristics of the nurse-client relationship have been elaborated upon in the foregoing discussion of goals, benefits, duration, and conditions as they would be operationalized in a nurse-client contract. We will now turn our attention to the last aspect of the relationship concept to be discussed in this chapter.

STAGES OF A RELATIONSHIP

As a person goes about his activities of daily living under normal circumstances, little thought is given to the manner in which relationships are established, maintained, or dissolved. However, nurses must purposefully establish, maintain, and dissolve their nurse-client relationships with a variety of people in many different settings. The nurse-client relationship usually takes place when the client's behavioral stability is already precarious. Since this relationship is the means by which the nurse assists the client to regain or maintain his steady state, its success can be enhanced when the process of each stage of the relationship is understood.

There is general agreement that a relationship can be divided into three stages or phases, although you may find that some people label the stages differently. The three stages are: (1) orientation, (2) utilization, and (3) resolution. Although these three stages are universal to any relationship, this discussion will concentrate on the nurse-client relationship.

There are two general points to be made before continuing with the discussion of each stage. First, the three stages are always sequential, but the stages cannot be limited to any specific time frame. Sometimes movement through one or all three stages is slow; other times the movement through one or all the stages is rapid. Movement through the stages can, at times, be so rapid that it may seem as though the stages occur simultaneously. Second, these three stages can also be identified in the process of each interaction within the relationship. Each contact with the client has an orientation phase that becomes increasingly brief as the relationship develops a utilization phase that becomes lengthened as the relationship continues, and a resolution stage as the interactional period is terminated.

The orientation stage

The orientation stage starts at the point of the initial interaction and continues until such time as there is a mutual understanding and acceptance of a relationship contract. In other words, during this stage the problems or reasons for the interaction are identified, the goals are established, the duration specified, the rights and obligations of the participants are defined, and their roles are clarified. The purpose of this stage is to provide a solid foundation for further interaction.

The most important outcome of this stage is the establishment of *trust* between the participants of the relationship. Trust is defined as a feeling of safety in sharing one's own thoughts and feelings with another. An individual will limit his information sharing in order to protect the integrity of his self-concept; he will be willing to share information about his thoughts and feelings only to the extent that he determines what is relevant and safe. The trust may be total if a person is willing to share thoughts and feelings about all aspects of his life with another person; however, it is to be expected that the trust will extend only to the area of information that the person believes appropriate to the nurse-client relationship.

This stage can be characterized as a "testing out" period for those involved. It is a fallacy to think that trust is automatically extended to the nurse just because a person assumes a client position and vice versa. During this time the client is deciding whether or not the nurse is actually a reliable helping person, and the nurse is determining the person's reliability as a client.

The orientation stage is also characterized by an exchange of information. Nurses are concerned not only with gathering data but also with giving information. There is some information that clients must share with nurses and some information that nurses must share with clients. It is too limiting to characterize the orientation stage as the data-gathering phase because it implies a one-way movement of information, client to nurse.

The nurse may require very personal and private information from the patient. In order to facilitate accurate exchange of information and enhance the feelings of trust, the nurse will often need to make the client aware of the reasons for questions of a personal nature. The client may be reluctant to answer unless he understands why the information is needed. Consequently, the nurse who gives a general explanation of why certain information is useful is more likely to elicit accurate responses from the patient and with less intensification of his stress state.

The process of information exchange that occurs during the orientation stage can also help to minimize many problems arising from preconceived ideas. Both the nurse and the client may make erroneous assumptions or rely on stereotyping when entering a new relationship. The structural variable profile with its two-step assessment is one tool that nurses can use during this phase to minimize their faulty assumptions and avoid the pitfalls of stereotyping (Chapter 4). The client may need help to disregard his erroneous assumptions, which may be based on preconceptions or lack of information. Some common assumptions that clients often make are: (1) hospitals are places where one goes to die; (2) orderlies and doctors are males; (3) nurses are females; (4) all injections are narcotic medications for pain; and (5) public health nurses are concerned only with "social diseases." Through the initial exchange of information nurses attempt to ensure that they themselves do not make unwarranted assumptions about the client and that the client has the knowledge that will enable him to disregard his faulty assumptions.

The information exchange should go beyond the data about the specific client and the particular nurse participating in the relationship. The client's understandings about the health functions of any agency or institution must be validated. The exchange must be extended to include information about the agency or institution the nurse represents so that the roles can be clarified in context with its health functions. Even though the general public has some knowledge of hospitals, the hospital setting is fraught with ambiguities, and a person can easily become perplexed and confused. The client and his family may be bewildered by the variety of hospital activities, instrumentation, and array of workers to which they are exposed. A variety of health team members wear white uniforms, caps, and pins; some registered nurses wear colored uniforms or street clothes; and monitoring and treatment equipment looks like something imported from outer space. Consequently, the nurse must specify the contributions made by the various team members, explain the equipment encountered, and indicate how activities of others will be related to those of the nurse and the client.

The general public is less well informed about the contributions that can be made by nursing personnel representing a variety of other agencies and institutions in the community, such as health departments, visiting nurse associations, schools, and industries. Nurses encountering families that have had no previous contact with the agency they represent must determine what knowledge the family has of the agency's health functions generally. For instance, it should not be surprising that many illegal aliens avoid contact with the health department nurses for fear of being reported for deportation. Some middle- and upper-class families consider the health department an agency that serves only the indigent population, and they are reluctant to utilize any of its services. A school nurse, making a home visit after notification by a teacher that a student had been absent 3 days because of "convulsions," was mistaken for a truant officer and received a negative reception until this misconception was clarified. Occupational health nurses, too, are often faced with similar situations. Consequently, the client and his family must understand the health contribution that can be made by the agency or the institution the nurse represents before the specific role can be understood and accepted.

The orientation stage is also characterized by repetition and reclarification of material previously introduced. The exchange often takes place during a period when a person's stress state has been intensified by an illness and additionally intensified because the person is still working through his transition into the client position. Therefore the individual may not hear or retain what is said, or may even distort that information shared. Since the client may be easily overwhelmed, the nurse must limit the information exchange to the degree to which it is useful to the client. The nurse must determine the amount, rate, and method that will enhance the information exchange so that the maximum benefits accrue with a minimum of stress intensification.

At the beginning of this section we indicated that it is impossible to establish a specific time allotment for completion of any one of the relationship stages. There are times when the nursing personnel may slip into the utilization stage with a minimum of time given to the orientation stage because of the nature of the understandings that both the client and the nurse have about the situation. For example, a 23-year-old man fell off a bicycle and was admitted into the emergency unit with his arm obviously broken. The understanding of the problem, expectations for action, rights, and obligations, and roles were rapidly clarified by the patient and nurse; trust was quickly established. Of course, if the fracture was complicated and surgery had been needed, or if other problems had been identified, the orientation stage might have been lengthened. There can be a great deal of variation in the time necessary to accomplish the purpose of this stage, depending upon the persons involved and their particular set of circumstances. However, if the utilization stage is to be efficient and productive, the orientation stage must have been successfully completed.

The utilization stage

The utilization stage is the period during which the nurse and the client are working together to achieve the goals established for their relationship. This stage is composed of a series of nurse-client interactions. Each interaction has short-term objectives that contribute in some way to the overall relationship goals. Just as with the relationship goals, the more definitive the short-term objectives, the easier they are to achieve with resulting feelings of accomplishment. Also, these objectives must be realistically related to the time allocated for their accomplishment.

Each interaction itself will have a brief orientation phase to review intervening events, to update information, and to agree upon the short-term objectives for the specified time allotment. Additionally, if the client's situation as altered drastically (improved or deteriorated), there may be a need to alter the relationship contract (goals, duration, or conditions) at this time. The "work" of each period is followed by a short resolution phase when the accomplishments of the work period are evaluated, objectives for the next interaction or series of interactions determined, any required interim activities identified, and the time of the next interaction tentatively or specifically established.

The utilization stage of a nurse-client relationship is characterized by interventions that reflect the nurse's concern for the person as a holistic being. The nurse continues to assist the client to modify his patterned behaviors when necessitated by the illness or potential illness and to support those behaviors that need not be disrupted; interventions during this period will revolve around helping the person to adjust his activities of daily living within the limitations imposed by any symptoms and treatments of the specific pathologic or potential pathologic conditions. Because of this holistic perspective, the nurse's interventions will be an amalgamation of those interventions that are undertaken as a result of the nursing knowledge and those interventions that have been delegated by the physician as a result of his diagnostic and treatment program.

This stage is also characterized by a "doing with" kind of intervention in which the client is considered an active participant in the process. It is crucial to the relationship that the individual *not* be considered a passive recipient of nursing care, regardless of his level of wellness. The practice of those nurses who view the client as a passive recipient is characterized by a "doing to" or "doing for" kind of interaction. Granted, a person may be in a dependent position, but he is still an active participant in all that happens to him and around him. Even the critically ill person thought to be unconscious should be considered as an active participant; he may hear although he is unable to respond. You may think it odd to observe a nurse communicating with an unconscious patient as if he might respond. It is a pleasant experience to elicit a response from a person not thought capable of a response, and it is an unpleasant experience to have a patient who regains consciousness tell you that he was distressed by the conversations about him when it was thought he could not hear. Furthermore, it must be remembered that the patient position is occupied temporarily. Even the person who may be left with residual disabilities will rarely occupy the dependent patient position forever. He should be encouraged to be as independent as possible within the limitations of his situation so that his attention will be focused on the strengths or positive aspects of his situation rather than be governed by the negative ones. The transition into and out of the client position will be accomplished with less stress intensification when nursing care is characterized by a "doing with" intervention.

The resolution stage

The resolution stage is the final or last period of a relationship. Resolution obviously includes the notions of termination or conclusion. However, it goes beyond this simple idea of an ending, because a relationship can be terminated without the resolution phase ever being incorporated into the process. Resolution occurs only when there is mutual agreement to end the relationship and the basis for the termination is acceptable.

Incorporation of the resolution phase helps ensure that there will be a minimum of stress intensification caused by the termination itself. Sometimes the participants will be happy to end a relationship especially if the client is vacating the client position because of an elevation in level of wellness. At other times, ending a relationship may be quite frightening to a person who has become accustomed to varying degrees of support from a particular nurse. The nurse, too, may be reluctant to terminate the relationship. The resolution stage enables both the nurse and client to achieve a sense of accomplishment and closure regardless of whether the client is actually vacating the client position or whether it is the nurse who must withdraw from their relationship.

The resolution stage is characterized by a joint nurse-client evaluation of the progress that has been made during their interaction periods compared with the goals established at the outset of their relationship. The discussion includes the following points: (1) the strengths or positive factors in the situation, (2) the weaknesses or areas that will need continuing effort on the part of the client in order to increase his level of wellness, and (3) the resources that are available to the client when this particular relationship has ended. Discussion of each of these factors should assist both the client and the nurse to understand the reasons for and accept the conclusion of their relationship.

The resolution stage is ultimately enhanced by the discussion of a time frame or expectation of duration that occurred during the orientation phase when the relationship contract was being established. The direct and early approach to the factor of time helps the client to limit his demands and expectations to those that can be realistically accomplished during their relationship so that termination is more readily accepted when those goals have been accomplished. The client usually is better prepared to enter the resolution phase if an arbitrary time limitation is known from the outset. For instance, an arbitrary time period may be imposed on the relationship because of the nurse's weekly work and vacation schedule. When the nurse must leave his case, the client may feel sad and experience a sense of loss; however, he will not have been deceived into thinking that he can depend on a particular nurse as long as he remains in the client position.

Sometimes a relationship will be terminated without incorporation of the resolution stage. This, hopefully, will occur infrequently and only when a relationship is ended without forewarning by circumstances beyond the control of either of the participants. For example, clients may be unexpectedly transferred from one unit to another or to another health agency, or may die. Similarly, nurses may be assigned without notice to a different unit or they even become ill themselves. In these situations both the client and the nurse may feel a sense of loss, a lack of accomplishment, or anger. The client may be left with feelings of rejection or desertion, and the nurse may feel guilty because he or she did not complete the work scheduled with the client.

The nurse must make a concerted effort to include the resolution phase into each nurse-client relationship. The phase need not be prolonged but must be incorporated so that feelings of accomplishment and closure can be achieved by all those participating in the relationship.

SUMMARY

The reciprocal designation of nurse and of client as counterpositions specifies the nature of the resulting relationship as professional; therefore the nurse-client relationship is governed by the stipulations of a professional relationship. A nurse and a client, however, may interact without their interactions culminating in a relationship if there is not mutual determination and acceptance of goal-directed activities.

Nurses will attempt to make a relationship contract as explicit as possible because it provides the ground rules for their interactions with the client. Nurses establish a relationship contract with their clients by reaching agreement on the specific health goals to be achieved, acknowledgment of benefits, determination of duration, and identification of the conditions that will govern their interactions. Each nurse-client contract will reflect the individual differences of the participants, within the parameters of a professional relationship. Nurses can facilitate the nurse-client relationship by purposefully incorporating an orientation, a utilization, and a resolution stage into each of their relationships.

To conclude, since the interactional process is the vehicle used by the nurse to assist a client in regaining or maintaining his steady state, the nurse must be consciously aware of the scope and limitations of the nurse-client relationship and of the stages that must be incorporated into every relationship. These understandings, when implemented in the various settings, will enhance the productivity of the nurse-client relationship.

REFERENCE

1. Stein, Jess: The Random House dictionary of the English Language, unabridged edition, New York, 1966, Random House, Inc.

ADDITIONAL READINGS

Burgess, A. W., and Lazare, Aaron: Psychiatric nursing in the hospital and the community, Englewood Cliffs, N.J., 1976, Prentice-Hall Inc., chap. 10.

Greenhill, M. H.: Interviewing with a purpose, American Journal of Nursing **56:**1259, 1956.

Peplau, Hildegard E.: Interpersonal relations in nursing, New York, 1952, G. P. Putnam's Sons.

Chapter 10

A FRAMEWORK FOR NURSING PRACTICE

The content presented in this book directs attention to the nursing profession's primary or central reason for existence as a separate professional entity. Emphasis is placed on the nurse's role in assisting the client to maximize his adaptive processes in daily living so that he will be able to function as effectively and efficiently as possible and to actualize himself according to his nature.

The very essence of nursing practice evolves because of the secondary problems caused by interference with the client's ability to carry on his customary daily living behaviors. These problems can critically influence the rate and kind of adjustments the person and his family will make to the disease process or during the cure process. Who, other than the nurse, is prepared to assist the client to make the totality of necessary adjustments in his daily life in support of *both* the underlying physiologic processes and his accommodations in the world in which he exists? Who, if the nurse ignores the secondary problems, is in a position to help the client to cope as a unified whole and as a member of a family? Assisting the client with these necessary adjustments is a very specific function of the nursing profession and provides a large portion of the nurse's reason for being.

The scientific knowledge explosion has had an impact on the practice of both the medical and nursing professions. In the past, because of a dearth of precise knowledge, a disease condition too often had to simply run its course. The individual either got well or he died, with very little real intervention in the process. Both the physician and the nurse were limited to simple supportive measures that, hopefully, assisted the person to combat his disease successfully. The advent of highly refined diagnostic techniques and effective treatments has now, however, enabled the medical profession to combat pathology more directly and aggressively. Many nurses who had worked closely with physicians have now found themselves swept along to the disease process emphasis also. This has been unfortunate because a disease pathology focus tends to deemphasize the importance of the problems secondary to the disease process, which in the past were necessarily the major and common concern of both the doctor and the nurse.

Before nursing students are ready to explore the responsibilities delegated to them by the doctor, it is essential that they first understand the principal reason for the very existence of a ''nurse.'' With the perspective provided in this book, it is hopefully clear to the reader that nursing can provide a vital and unduplicated contribution to the welfare of the client. The nurse does not exist simply to serve the physician, even though an important part of his or her function is assisting the doctor by assuming delegated medical responsibilities. Neither does the nurse exist to diagnose a pathologic condition or prescribe treatment, even though under some circumstances the nursing role may be extended to include diagnosis and treatment of psychophysiopathology.*

Similar to the physician's dilemma in the past, nurses, too, worked from a very limited scientific base of knowledge. The current status of the behavioral and natural sciences, combined with improved methods of instruction in the nursing process now, however, provide the nurse with a much stronger knowledge base on which to assess and predict organismic behavioral responses in all health settings.

The key concepts selected for introductory study in this book provide a frame of reference for both the study and practice of nursing in its most fundamental sense. The contribution that the concepts make to this frame of reference is summarized in the following paragraphs.

The *organismic behavior concept* places the emphasis on the whole Man responding as a unified system. It directs the nurse to take into account a web of variables rather than considering particular behaviors as isolated happenings. Within this frame of reference, Man is conceptualized as a biopsychosocial energy unit consisting of a set of open subsystems and existing as an open system in his universe.

The *steady state concept* emphasizes that the individual strives both to maintain an internal constancy and to be in harmony with his external world. Neither the automatic physiochemical regulatory processes alone nor the voluntary and deliberative behaviors alone will maintain the steady state. Only the total effect of their combined efforts results in its maintenance, freeing the individual to actualize himself according to his nature.

The *concept of basic human needs* provides a basis for understanding the behaviors of Man, a holistic biopsychosocial being, as he goes about his activities of daily living. It directs attention to seven needs viewed on an equal par whose requirements can become motivating forces impelling behavior at various behavioral levels. It enables the nurse to understand and anticipate both automatic psychochemical regulatory processes and voluntary self-regulating behavior that may lead to goal

---

*The nurse midwife, the pediatric nurse practitioner, and the nurse who works in a crisis intervention center are examples of the expanded role of the nurse. Chapters 7 and 8 in *Current Perspectives in Nursing* may be helpful to the reader who is curious about the expanded role of the nurse.[1,2]

achievement when need imbalances are perceived. Moreover, it directs the nurse to consider the interrelationships between the needs by continually focusing attention on their combined effect as a person carries out his ordinary activities.

The *adaptation concept* refers to the constructive end results that occur when adjustments are made to either internal or external changes affecting the person as an ongoing functioning unit. There are some behaviors that will be adaptive in nature and others that will be maladaptive. This concept impels the nurse to examine the nature of the adjustments made in terms of Man as an integrated behavioral unit and the implications his current adjustments will have for his ability to function as a whole in the future.

The *behavioral patterning concept,* an an adaptive process employed by Man, enables the nurse to comprehend more fully the impact that the illness situation will have on the patient and how he can be assisted to adjust his activities of daily living to meet the demands of the illness situation.

The *structural variable concept* directs the nurse's attention to a set of factors, each factor representing a category of generalizations that can be drawn upon to understand people who share similar characteristics, traits, and beliefs. The concept directs the nurse to establish a client's profile, undertaking a two-step assessment process. The nurse is directed to (1) identify all the appropriate generalizations that correspond to each particular profile factor of that client and then (2) determine the degree to which the generalizations actually govern or influence that client's behavioral responses. This assessment will help the nurse in understanding and anticipating how a person may respond in the illness situation.

The *level of wellness concept* provides a health continuum whereby the nurse will focus on the positive attributes and characteristics of a client within the dimensions of his situation.

The *stress concept* has been used to indicate a state that is always present but that is intensified when there is a change or a threat with which the individual must cope. When it becomes intensified, it will usually exceed the limits of the steady state, and in this case the person will be using more than the usual amount of energy in his attempt to adapt. Moderate intensification of the stress state is essential for growth and learning, while an excessive degree of intensification is usually maladaptive. When the stress state intensifies, nurses will be able to identify observable changes in a person's features and actions; they will observe and evaluate changes in both the voluntary self-regulatory behaviors and behavioral changes that reflect an alteration in automatic physiologic activity. Nurses will be concerned with an imbalance between the demands made by the internal or external environments and the responsive capacities of the client. They will focus on the daily living adjustments necessary to prevent illness or enhance the healing process.

The *behavioral stability continuum concept* evolves from the steady state and stress concepts and provides the nurse with a method of assessing the appropriateness of the client's allocation of his energies and his potential for utilizing his adaptive capacities. The effectiveness and efficiency of the client's behavior can be assessed with considerable objectivity by careful examination of the consistency, coherency, and orderliness of his behaviors as an integrated behavioral unit.

"An act has more than one consequence" concept has been used to focus the nurse's attention on the outcomes to be achieved by nursing intervention. The full scope of the contribution that the nurse can make will be evident when this concept becomes a part of the nurse's thought process.

The interrelated *concepts of position and role* provide the nurse with a means of systematically examining the rights and obligations of various positions and complementary counterpositions and of examining the behaviors that meaningfully and appropriately constitute the role attached to a position. These concepts direct the nurse's attention to the confusion and conflict that occurs when there is a difference between behavioral expectations and role enactment.

The *concept of a relationship* directs attention to the specific nature of the relationship existing between a nurse and a client. It emphasizes the necessity for an explicit relationship contract that stipulates the parameters of the nurse-client relationship, which is a professional type of relationship. The concept also directs attention to the stages of a relationship that must be incorporated during any nurse-client relationship so that it will be both efficient and effective.

The translation of these concepts into workable forces can be accomplished in several ways. We suggest that the transition between theoretical generalizations and clinical application can be achieved by posing a series of questions to be answered. The questions must be valid if the students and practitioners are to gather the kind of data essential to their practice. Moreover, if the questions are ordered properly, the progressive accumulation of data should enable them to reach some very constructive conclusions on which to base their nursing intervention.

The questions that follow evolved through the beginning study of the concepts that have been presented; they have been raised with no attempt to answer them here. Their usefulness will be validated when they are utilized in the clinical setting in conjunction with both the nursing and psychophysiopathology content to be presented in other texts and courses. These questions can be grouped under seven major headings.*

A. Questions that will determine the particular structural variable profile for each person involved in the situation:
   1. What are the specific characteristics of each profile factor?
      a. What is their age and sex?
      b. What is their ethnic and cultural background?

---

*What may appear as duplication of some of the questions occurs to ensure that the patient situation is viewed from all perspectives.

 c. What is their religious affiliation?
 d. What is their educational and occupational background?
 e. Who are the "significant others" involved?
 f. What is their health status?
 2. What are the generalizations that might be relevant to a person with the characteristics of this profile?
 3. To what degree do the identified generalizations actually influence or govern the person's behavior in this situation?
B. Questions that identify potential problems and potential resources:
 1. What are the limitations with which the client must cope?
 2. How does the client view his situation?
 a. What priority does the client give to his human needs?
 b. Does he have only a here-and-now orientation?
 c. Is he seeing himself as a unified whole or only as his involved part?
 d. How does the individual view or evaluate his potential capacity?
 3. To what degree is he utilizing the potential of which he is capable?
 4. What are the behaviors composing the client's usual patterns of daily living?
 5. What are the disruptions in his usual behaviors caused by the illness situation?
 6. Within the limits of the medical regimen, which of the disruptions in his behavioral patterns are actually necessary?
 7. What are the external environmental resources available to him? How can they be utilized more effectively?
C. Questions that give an indication of the client's adaptation status, the appropriateness of his energy allocation, and his potential adaptive capacity:
 1. Is the client's behavioral adjustment adaptive or maladaptive?
 2. What is the client's position on the behavioral stability continuum?
 a. Are his behaviors effective and efficient, or effective but not efficient or vice versa, or neither effective nor efficient?
 b. To what degree are his behaviors consistent, coherent, and orderly?
 c. Are there any behavioral cues that may indicate intensification of the stress state in the following categories:
 (1) Accentuated use of some usual mode or pattern of behavior?
 (2) Alteration in the variety of activities usually undertaken?
 (3) Less organized behavior or a lower level of behavioral organization?
 (4) Demonstration of greater sensitivity to the environment?
 (5) Presence of behaviors reflecting alteration in his ordinary subsystem activity?
 (6) Distortion of "reality"?

D. Questions that give an indication of the client's ability to utilize his adaptive capacity constructively including the factors that affect his ability to change:
   1. Do both the nurse and the client give the same priority in the ranking of the client's basic human needs in the specific illness situation?
   2. What is the status of the stressors for a particular situation?
      a. What is the nature of the stressor?
      b. How many stressors must be coped with simultaneously?
      c. How long has or will the client be exposed to the stressor?
      d. What has been his previous experience with a comparable stressor?
   3. How successfully can the client be motivated to change his behavior?
      a. What is the source of the stimuli?
      b. What is the intensity or number of the stimuli?
      c. What is the specific behavior or pattern of behavior involved?
      d. What importance does the client attach to the original behavior?
E. Questions that will identify nursing intervention that will be required:
   1. For whom does this particular activity have consequences?
   2. What are the consequences that can be anticipated?
   3. What is the value of those consequences for those involved?
F. Questions that will give an indication of the effectiveness of the nurse-client interactional process will have two directions:
   1. Questions of the client that may indicate stressors or potential stressors:
      a. What does the person view as his rights and obligations in the client position?
      b. What is his understanding of the client role behaviors and the behaviors of the nurse role?
      c. Can confusion or conflict between roles attached to his other positions and that of the client role be anticipated under the prevailing circumstances?
      d. Does the client understand and accept the ground rules of this nurse-client relationship?
   2. Questions that nurses must ask themselves:
      a. Do the client's understandings of his role and the nurse role differ from my understandings in this situation?
      b. Have I clarified the ground rules of this professional relationship in my own mind?
      c. Are all the stages of a relationship being fully incorporated in my interactions with a given patient?
      d. Am I appropriately enacting the nurse role in this situation?
      e. Do I inadvertently shift roles when the nurse position is the governing position?

    f. Are there conflicting demands of other positions I occupy that influence my enactment of the nurse role?

G. Questions that nurses must continually ask of themselves so that their practice will continue to reflect the highest level of professional competence:

    1. Am I fulfilling the full scope of my professional obligations in my daily practice?

    2. Are my rights as a professional nurse being acknowledged in such a way that I can best fulfill my professional obligations?

    3. To what degree am I depending upon external rules and regulations to govern my actions?

    4. Am I using discrimination when I delegate tasks to other categories of health workers or family members?

    5. Am I judicious in accepting tasks delegated to me?

All of these questions should become an integral part of the nurse practitioner's thought processes. The nurse who consistently considers these questions will not lose sight of the vital and fundamental contribution that can be made through nurse-client interaction.

The approach to nursing and the content presented in this book are but a basic framework into which the student must add the many additional theories and facts that are presented in the various courses that constitute the still evolving science of nursing. This framework is functional and appropriate for nursing intervention in any setting. Clients can be assisted to attain and maintain their highest level of wellness whether they are encountered in a hospital, doctor's office, or clinic or on a home visit, to name but a few of the places where nursing care may be given.

In this current time when expansion of the parameters of the nurse's responsibilities are compounding, we submit that such a framework becomes even more essential. With primary care based on the conceptual basis suggested in this text, the nurse can easily assume additional responsibilities without loss of his or her basic vital and unduplicated contribution to the welfare of the recipient of health care.

REFERENCES

1. Henshaw, S. K.: The nurse practitioner movement. In Miller, M. H., and Flynn, B. C.: Current perspectives in nursing: social issues and trends, St. Louis, 1977, The C. V. Mosby Co., pp. 80-92.
2. Gage, L. W.: Partners in primary care. In Miller, M. H., and Flynn, B. C.: Current perspectives in nursing; social issues and trends, St. Louis, 1977, The C. V. Mosby Co., pp. 94-101.

ADDITIONAL READINGS

Cherescavich, Gertrude: Open forum: shortage or misuse of professional nursing skills, Nursing Forum **9**(3):224-234, 1970.

Christman, Luther: What the future holds for nursing, Nursing Forum **9**(1):12-18, 1970.

Lysaught, J. P., director: An abstract for action, New York, 1970, McGraw-Hill Book Co.

Murphy, Juanita F.: Role expansion or role extension: some conceptual differences, Nursing Forum **9**(4):380-390, 1970.

GLOSSARY OF TERMS

activities of daily living Those customary activities, both essential and basic in everyone's day, such as eating, eliminating, sleeping, working, and socializing.

adaptation The positive, constructive end results that occur for the person as an ongoing functioning unit when adjustments are made to either an internal or an external environmental change.

adaptive energy That energy that is consumed as Man adapts to a stressor.

allocation To distribute a fixed amount; to set apart for a specific purpose.

antagonistic Acting in opposition to.

assess To estimate or determine the significance, importance, or value of.

atomistic Made up of a number of unrelated elements.

atrophy Wasting away of a body tissue or organ.

behavior A response to stimuli. Since this term is a broad, all-inclusive term, the behavioral level or focal unit to be analyzed must be identified (see organismic behavior).

behavioral features Observable characteristics of the physical shell housing Man.

behavioral norms The designated standards of average performance of people of a given age, background, and so on.

behavioral pattern A cluster of behaviors that appear to have a common drive or goal; distribution of habitually used behaviors occurring in such a way that a design evolves.

behavioral stability The ability of Man to maintain or reestablish the steady state when it has been disrupted by either internal or external stressors.

client A consumer of health care service; a person who is actively engaged, regardless of where he is on the health continuum, in attaining or maintaining a high level of wellness.

closed system System that is self-contained, totally isolated and, therefore, not affected by changes outside its boundaries.

cognitive processes Those mental activities of knowing in the broad sense, including perception, judgment, and memory.

coherency The quality of being consistent; logically integrated.

concept The label of a set of things or ideas classified at a level of generality that will permit use of the notion or idea in relation to a wide variety of situations that go together.

consistency Agreement; harmony; logical connection.

continuum A continuous whole whose parts cannot be separated or separately discerned.

cope To deal with problems; to contend with successfully.

covert Concealed, hidden, or disguised.

crisis Any unusual, extreme, or threatening situation that calls for immediate resolution of the stressors or reallocation of energies so that adaptation can occur.

deliberate behavior Those organismic responses of man occurring as a result of his thought processes; voluntary rather than automatic reflex behaviors.

dichotomize To divide or separate into two parts.

environment All the conditions, circumstances, and influences surrounding and affecting the organism.

142

feedback mechanisms A process by which the factors that produce a result are themselves modified, corrected, or strengthened by that result.

holistic The view that an integrated whole has a reality independent of and greater than the sum of its parts.

homeostasis The maintenance of internal stability in an organism by coordinated responses of the organ systems that automatically compensate for environmental changes.

homeostatic mechanisms The automatic physiologic regulatory mechanisms that tend to maintain internal constancy.

individual norms The designated expectations of a specific individual's performance based upon his usual performance under his ordinary circumstances.

integrity The quality or state of being complete, unimpaired, sound.

internal constancy A state of physiologic stability in which the organism by coordinated response of the body systems compensates for environmental changes.

maladaptation Nonconstructive or destructive consequences that occur for Man as an ongoing functioning unit when adjustments are made to either an internal or external environmental change.

observations Information collected through the use of Man's five senses: auditory, gustatory, olfactory, tactile, and visual.

open system One that is directly affected by happenings or changes in other systems in its environment.

optimal tension level That level at which Man has achieved a balance between utilization and conservation of his energy.

organismic behavior Those observable features and actions that reflect Man's functioning as a unified whole within the environment in which he exists.

overt Open, observable, apparent, not hidden.

palliative Affording relief but not cure.

parameter A quantity to which the operator may assign arbitrary values; in this text, used to refer to the arbitrary outer limits or boundaries of a function or situation.

pathology The functional and structural changes in the body that cause or are caused by disease.

patient A person who has placed himself under medical or surgical treatment.

perception A psychologic experience in which sensory stimuli are integrated to form an image, the significance of which is influenced by past experiences.

population norms The designated expectations of average performance of Man as a species.

position The social identity assigned a particular location in social space.

role A collection of behaviors thought to constitute a meaningful unit and deemed appropriate to a person occupying a particular position.

significant others Those other persons whose relationship has a specific meaning. ''Significant others'' may include family or nonfamily members and the relationship may be characterized as either a primary or a secondary relationship.

steady state That state existing when Man is allocating his energy in such a way that he is freed to actualize himself according to his nature, maintained by effective and efficient activities of the regulatory processes at all levels.

stress A state that is always present in Man but that is intensified when there is a change or threat with which the individual must cope.

stressor The factor or agent causing an intensification of the stress state.

synergistic The simultaneous action of separate factors that, together, have greater total effect than the sum of their individual effects.

system A whole that functions as a whole by virtue of the interdependence of its parts.

tension A state of strain, tautness.

INDEX